Nutrition Assistant Essentials

Barbara Acello

THOMSON
DELMAR LEARNING

Australia Canada Mexico Singapore Spain United Kingdom United States

THOMSON
DELMAR LEARNING

Nutrition Assistant Essentials
by Barbara Acello

Vice President, Health Care Business Unit:
William Brottmiller

Editorial Director:
Cathy L. Esperti

Acquisitions Editor:
Marah Bellegarde

Marketing Director:
Jennifer McAvey

Marketing Coordinator:
Michele Gleason

Senior Production Editor:
James Zayicek

Printed in the United States of America.
1 2 3 4 5 6 7 XXX 08 07 06 05 04

For more information, contact Thomson Delmar Learning, 5 Maxwell Drive, Clifton Park, NY 12065

Or find us on the World Wide Web at http://www.delmarlearning.com

Library of Congress Cataloging-in-Publication Data

ISBN 1-4018-7211-5

CONTENTS

PREFACE

Nutrition Assistant Essentials is designed to prepare the nutrition assistant to work in a long-term care facility, hospital skilled unit, subacute care center, or other long-term care setting. The text emphasizes "real-world" practice, and provides solutions to common problems that nutrition assistants may encounter. Compliance with current infection control and safety practices as well as state and federal regulations is highlighted.

Over the years, the acuity of residents in long-term care facilities has increased markedly. Residents of the twenty-first century are much sicker and more dependent on staff for care. The nursing assistant profession has also evolved from an unlicensed, untrained workforce to a group of educated, skilled paraprofessionals who pass a certification examination and are listed with the state nursing assistant registry. More is expected of nursing assistants than ever before in the history of long-term care. Mealtime is especially challenging. Many residents require assistance. Passing trays, assisting residents with meals, and documenting intake is time-consuming. Ensuring residents receive food that is appetizing and served at the proper temperature is no small feat.

In 2003, the federal government passed Medicare and Medicaid Programs; Requirements for Paid Feeding Assistants in Long Term Care Facilities 42 CFR Parts 483 and 488 [CMS–2131–F]. This law gives states the authority to use paid, noncertified assistants to help with meal service in long-term care facilities. These individuals are permitted to assist only those residents with basic, uncomplicated feeding needs. They must work under the remote (indirect) supervision of a licensed nurse. State agencies must establish criteria for teaching and employing nutrition (feeding) assistants in their state. These employees may be staff from non-nursing departments. They may also be hired specifically to assist residents during meals. The requirement does not apply to volunteers or residents' family members.

The federal law specifies that these individuals have a minimum of eight hours of education in assisting residents with nutrition and hydration, feeding techniques, communication, responding to resident behavior, resident rights, safety and emergencies, infection control, and recognizing and reporting changes in residents' conditions. States have the flexibility of requiring more than the minimum number of hours of preparation. They have the authority to set criteria for who may offer classes and to establish instructor qualifications.

Nutrition Assistant Essentials is designed to parallel the required curriculum for these workers. There is no "universal curriculum" for nutrition assistant education. We have grouped common and required subjects together in logical order. The main focus is on clinical practice. Theory is included when it is necessary to understand the reason for a procedure or to apply the information to other similar situations.

ORGANIZATION

Our goal in developing this book was to provide "one-stop shopping" for the nutrition assistant and instructor. The book is designed to be all-inclusive, without the need for additional supplements.

- Objectives are included at the beginning of each chapter that highlight the important concepts being discussed.
- Step-by-step procedures clearly outline how to perform each skill.
- A review section is included at the end of each chapter that contains questions for homework or self-testing, to ensure the student masters the material.
- Procedure checklists can be found in the back of the book to be used as an assessment or self-check.

INSTRUCTOR RESOURCES

A companion instructor's manual provides

- resources for effective teaching
- critical thinking activities
- quizzes
- final examination

In the author's opinion, the resident is the most important individual in the long-term care facility. All care is directed to providing the highest quality of life possible for facility residents. Properly trained and motivated nutrition assistants are important for the well-being of residents and the overall operation of the long-term care facility. The addition of these workers will undoubtedly improve quality of life. The staff at Thomson Delmar Learning is committed to helping you succeed by providing quality educational materials to prepare you for your important responsibilities in the long-term health care delivery system.

ACKNOWLEDGMENTS

The author wishes to thank Marah Bellegarde, Acquisitions Editor of Thomson Delmar Learning, for her responsiveness to the needs of long-term care workers. Many individuals work behind the scenes at Delmar to ensure the project moves forward painlessly. Thank you all for your long hours, for your dedication and commitment to long-term care workers, and for making yourselves available.

A team of peer reviewers dropped everything and reviewed this book immediately after the federal law was passed. They have provided many helpful comments and given us all insight into the needs of workers in their states. Your input was invaluable, and I sincerely appreciate your cooperation and dedication.

Susan Lewsen, MA, BSN, RN
Davis Applied Technology College
Kaysville, UT

Margaret Konieczny, RN, MSN
Western Nevada Community College
Carson City, NV

Cissi Oloomi, MSN, RN, CNS, FNP, CNRN, CRRN-A
The Institute for Rehabilitation and Research (TIRR)
Houston, TX

Julie Slack, RN, MS, PhD (ABD)
Mohave Community College
Kingman, AZ

Lois Stotter, BSN, RNC
Patient Care Associate Program
Borgess Medical Center
Kalamazoo, MI

Linda Sullivan, MS, RN
Kansas City Community College
Kansas City, MO

UNIT 1

The Long-Term Care Facility

OBJECTIVES

- Spell and define key terms.
- Describe the types of residents admitted to the long-term care facility.
- State the purpose of the OBRA legislation.
- Explain why mealtime is a busy time in the long-term care facility.
- List some responsibilities of the nutrition assistant.
- Describe responsible behavior and list nine examples of ways to show that you are responsible.

THE LONG-TERM CARE FACILITY

Long-term care facilities offer many services. Some provide general care, while others focus on specialized services. Skilled nursing units in hospitals must follow the same laws as long-term care facilities. To be admitted to a long-term care facility, residents should be medically stable. If they are very ill, admission to the hospital may be more appropriate. Long-term care facilities are home to many types of residents. Most need help or supervision with daily self-care skills (Figure 1-1). Facility residents are not all elderly. Persons of all ages may be admitted. Some states require specially licensed facilities to care for infants and children. These facilities must arrange for the children's education. Some residents will spend the rest of their lives in the facility.

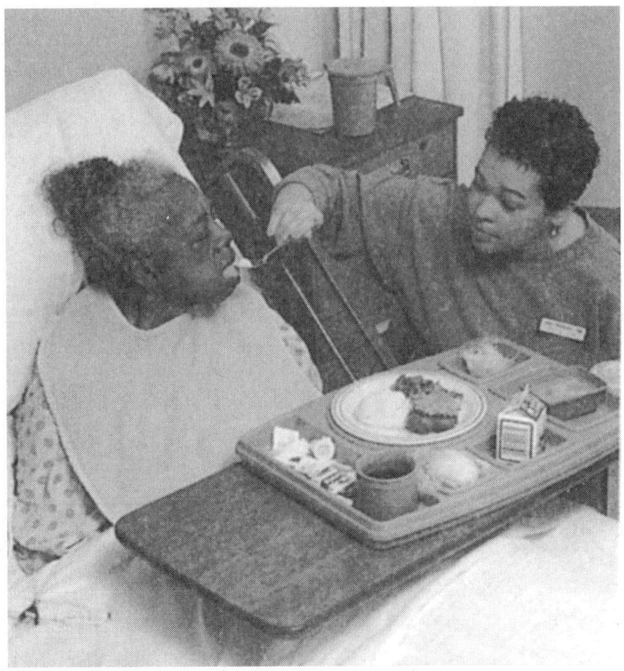

FIGURE 1-1
Most residents are admitted to the long-term care facility because they need assistance in meeting their daily personal and hygienic needs.

Others come to the facility for a short time, then return home. If younger residents are accepted, facilities usually must adapt their activity programs and menus to meet their needs. Young and middle-aged residents have different food preferences than most elderly individuals. They often enjoy fast foods, and food items such as stir fry, egg rolls, cheeseburgers, french fries, and tacos. Helping residents achieve the highest qualify of life possible is important. Providing nutritious food that looks and tastes good helps maintain quality of life.

Long-term care facilities are regulated and inspected by government agencies. They must follow state and federal laws for resident care, cleanliness, and safety. **OBRA** is the abbreviation for Omnibus Budget Reconciliation Act. The OBRA legislation of 1987 governs long-term care. These laws were designed to:

- improve residents' quality of life, quality of care, health, and safety
- provide a homelike environment
- maintain or improve residents' conditions
- promote independence

Being independent promotes healthy self-esteem. A plan of care is designed for each resident to assist that person to function at the highest level possible, considering her or his medical problems and needs. All workers caring for the resident must follow the care plan. This is an essential part of the OBRA philosophy.

Long-Term Care Facility Workers

Facilities must hire personnel with certain qualifications. Most direct personal care is provided by **nursing assistants**. The OBRA legislation sets minimum standards that all states must follow to ensure that nursing assistants are qualified to give personal care. The nursing assistant is an important member of the health care team. He or she spends more time with residents than any other caregiver. To work in a facility, the assistant must complete a state-approved program. The minimum required program length is 75 hours, but some nursing assistants have completed programs lasting several hundred hours. The nursing assistant must pass state written and competency (hands-on skills) examinations. The assistant is entered into the state nursing assistant registry. To keep certification active, he or she must work in health care and attend continuing education classes.

The nursing assistant is supervised by a licensed nurse. Long-term care facilities employ both **registered nurses (RNs)**, and **licensed practical nurses (LPNs)**. In Texas and California, these nurses are called **licensed vocational nurses (LVNs)**. An RN has completed two to four years of nursing education and has passed a state licensing examination. LPNs and LVNs have completed one year to 18 months of full-time nursing education and have passed a state licensing examination.

The health care industry needs many educated, qualified workers. The nursing department positions all require education and state testing, licensure, or certification. Inexperienced workers cannot be hired off the street and put immediately to work caring for residents. A nationwide shortage of health care workers began during the 1990s. Today the demand for health care workers exceeds the supply. At the same time, the need for long-term care facility services has never been as great. Because of this, facilities are exploring new ways of meeting the residents' needs with the staff available.

PROVIDING FOOD SERVICE AND MEALTIME ASSISTANCE

Good nutrition is essential for good health. The body must be well nourished to function properly and heal itself. Residents' height and weight are obtained on admission, and then weight is measured monthly or more often thereafter. A registered dietitian uses the weight, height, and other information to evaluate residents' nutritional needs. He or she writes the facility menus to ensure all residents receive a well-balanced diet. The dietitian also makes recommendations for meeting residents' medical needs, such as pressure ulcer treatment or diabetes management.

The dietary department prepares the meals. Nursing personnel are responsible for ensuring that residents receive food and fluids. In addition to delivering meals, staff must prepare trays by removing wrappers, cutting meat, buttering bread, opening milk cartons, providing straws, seasoning food, and so forth. They must verbally prompt some residents to eat. Staff refill beverages, and provide substitutes for foods if requested by a resident. In between meals, staff provide special supplements, nourishments, and snacks to some residents. They provide fresh drinking water and encourage and assist residents to drink enough liquid. Many residents must be spoon-fed and assisted in drinking liquids. OBRA permits only certain licensed and certified employees to feed residents and provide assistance with fluids.

Nutrition Assistants

As you can see, good nutrition and hydration are important for residents. To ensure good intake and prevent complications, facilities must create a pleasant, positive dining atmosphere for residents. Mealtimes are busy and time-consuming. Many residents need mealtime assistance. Foods must be served promptly to maintain the proper temperature. Maintaining food temperature helps prevent bacterial growth. Also, residents are most likely to accept foods of the proper temperature. No one likes to eat hot foods cold or cold foods hot! Unfortunately, staff shortages may make it difficult for facilities to meet residents' nutritional needs. Because of this, the federal government revised the law in 2003 to permit facilities to use nutrition assistants.

A **nutrition assistant** is a worker who has successfully completed a state-approved class. He or she may assist *certain residents* with food and fluids. Other titles for this position are:

- food and hydration aide or assistant
- nourishment aide or assistant
- nutritional aide
- nutrition/hydration assistant
- feeding assistant, feeding specialist, or feeding technician
- dining assistant, meal assistant, or resident assistant

The federal law requires a minimum of eight hours of education to work as a nutrition assistant. However, facilities or states may exceed the minimum requirements. The assistant must successfully complete the course before working with residents. Nutrition assistants are permitted to feed stable residents under the direction of a licensed nurse. Since residents' conditions sometimes change, your assignment may vary from day to day. Your facility will provide guidelines. Do not exceed the scope of your responsibility. Follow your job description, facility policies, and laws of your state. Some facilities assign additional tasks to this worker that do not involve direct care. An example job description is provided in Box 1-1. This job description lists a wide variety of responsibilities to give you an idea of the types of duties that may be assigned to the nutrition assistant. A nutrition assistant may:

- escort residents to the dining room
- serve and prepare food for residents
- prompt and encourage residents to eat, if necessary
- spoon-feed certain residents

BOX 1-1
Nutrition Assistant Job Description

Title: Nutrition assistant

Department: Nursing Service

Overview: A member of the resident care team who assists residents and staff with meal service, nutrition, and hydration as directed by a licensed nurse. Assists residents without complicated feeding problems in meeting their food and fluid needs.

Supervision: Works under the supervision of a registered nurse (RN) or licensed practical nurse (LPN)/licensed vocational nurse (LVN).

Knowledge, Skills, and Abilities
- sincerely likes and believes in people
- is considerate and understanding to residents, visitors, and other staff members
- follows directions, and functions according to expectations
- provides quality care, following the nurses' instructions according to RN directions and the resident's care plan
- proficient in documentation for assigned procedures

Language Skills: Ability to follow oral and written instructions in the English language

Reasoning Ability:
- able to follow directions
- is self-directed
- good interpersonal and communication skills with residents and co-workers
- able to use a hand-held calculator

Mathematical Skills:
Ability to complete simple calculations on a hand-held calculator.

Previous Experience:
No experience necessary.

Educational Requirements:
Successful completion of state-approved nutrition assistant program that includes at least the following minimum content:

(1) feeding techniques
(2) assistance with feeding and hydration
(3) communication and interpersonal skills
(4) appropriate responses to resident behavior
(5) safety and emergency procedures, including the Heimlich maneuver and how to get help in an emergency
(6) infection control
(7) resident rights
(8) recognizing changes in residents that are inconsistent with their normal behavior and the importance of reporting those changes to the supervisory nurse
- completion of a clinical externship/practicum, as required
- attends inservice and other educational programs and meetings, as required
- completion of a cardiopulmonary resuscitation (CPR) class is recommended, but not required (Hiring preference may be given to applicants with current CPR cards.)

BOX 1-1 *(continued)*

Physical Demands:
The physical demands listed here are representative of those that must be met by an employee to successfully perform the essential functions of this job. *Reasonable accommodations may be made to enable individuals with disabilities to perform the essential function.*

- able to stand, walk, and carry 5 pounds
- able to stoop and lift 5 pounds, using good body mechanics
- able to push equipment

Working Conditions:
The work environment characteristics described here are representative of those an employee encounters while performing the essential functions of this job. *Reasonable accommodations may be made to enable individuals with disabilities to perform the essential functions.* Long-term care facility employees may be exposed to infectious disease. Risk for harm is limited if the employee follows all infection control procedures and agency policies.

Essential Duties and Responsibilities
Performs technical procedures and routine dining tasks under the supervision of a licensed nurse including:

(1) Serves meal trays to residents.
  - Checks items on the tray to make sure they are allowed on the resident's diet.
  - Serves meals promptly so foods are at the proper temperature; checks food temperature by dropping a small amount on wrist.
  - Honors food preferences, likes, and dislikes.
  - Provides substitutes for meat and vegetables, according to facility policy.
  - Passes the dessert cart and offers residents a choice of items.

(2) Provides beverages and condiments.
  - Refills beverages, as requested.
  - Encourages fluids according to residents' individual care plans.

(3) Assists with resident tray preparation, including but not limited to cutting meat, opening milk cartons, providing straws, and buttering bread.

(4) Provides mealtime assistance as needed by residents, considering resident needs for independence and the nutritional plan of care.

(5) Speaks with residents, prompts and encourages residents to eat.
  - Prompts and cues the resident, if necessary, according to the care plan.
  - Before feeding residents, uses hand-over-hand technique in accordance with the care plan.
  - Allows enough time for residents to finish eating; avoids rushing.

(6) Feeds assigned residents.
  - Helps residents who are having trouble feeding themselves.
  - Provides adaptive utensils and dishes, according to the care plan.
  - Reheats cold food items, if necessary.

(7) Records food intake.

(8) Records fluid intake, as assigned.

(9) Tallies, trends, and documents residents' food and fluid intake records, as directed.

(10) Delivers fluids and snacks to residents twice daily, using the beverage cart and fruit basket.

(11) Serves, assists, and prompts residents to consume planned, ordered snacks and supplements.

(continues)

BOX 1-1 *(continued)*

(12) Informs nurse, dietary services manager, registered dietitian, or diet technician of any food and/or fluid intake problems, expressed likes and dislikes, as appropriate.
- Notifies nurse if a resident has difficulty feeding himself, eating, drinking, or using utensils.

(13) Uses good communication skills regarding individual resident needs, likes, dislikes, and abilities, participates in developing nutrition/hydration plan of care, as requested.

(14) Uses good observational skills, reports changes in the resident's self-feeding ability, appetite, and eating patterns to the nurse, recognizes and reports other observations and changes in residents' conditions and signs of acute illness to the nurse.

(15) Other responsibilities may include, but are not necessarily limited to:
- walking with residents and assisting them to their dining table
- assisting and escorting ambulatory and wheelchair-bound residents from their rooms to the dining area
- positioning and moving wheelchairs so exit pathways are clear
- observing residents for positioning problems for eating, including table too high, too low, too far away, etc., reports problems to nurse
- checking and logging food temperature on a "test tray" each day: hot food items should be at least 140 degrees F; Cold items should be 40 degrees F or cooler
- stocking and pushing the snack and hydration cart twice daily
- serving beverages to residents who are independent or who need only supervision or limited assistance to consume beverages
- Informing the nurse if a resident requires extensive assistance
- recording hydration cart fluid intake daily for residents on *"Intake Watch,"* calorie count, and/or intake and output monitoring
- maintaining an orderly, tidy work area by following all infection control precautions, emptying trash, and cleaning equipment, supplies, and work areas as assigned
- clearing, washing, and setting tables, as required
- assisting in decorating the dining room for holidays and special events
- assisting with "happy hour" on Fridays, by passing hors d'oeuvres and nonalcoholic beverages of residents' choice
- assisting residents in wiping faces and hands, removing clothing protectors and spilled food before leaving dining room
- supervising resident smoking in designated area after meals
- passing the "shopping cart" so residents may purchase items such as puzzle books and cheese crackers
- assisting residents with food and fluids during activities and special events, such as the ice cream social, pizza and birthday parties
- stocking the unit pantries each day
- monitoring and logging pantry refrigerator/freezer temperatures each day (Refrigerators should not exceed 40 degrees F.)
- making sure items stored in pantry refrigerators are covered, labeled, and dated
- checking the expiration date of packaged items in the pantry refrigerator, such as supplements and milk, discarding those that are beyond the expiration date
- discarding perishable items in pantry refrigerators according to facility policy (four days for cooked items, seven days for other packaged items) (Sealed items, such as cans of soda pop, may be refrigerated indefinitely and should not be discarded.)
- defrosting and cleaning pantry refrigerators according to posted schedule.

BOX 1-1 *(continued)*

(16) Works as a team member, assisting and providing support as needed.
(17) Meets resident needs or reports to the appropriate team member.
(18) Applies principles of infection control and good handwashing, uses alcohol-based hand cleansers according to facility policy.
(19) Restocks supplies and equipment, as needed.
(20) Follows all safety policies and procedures; reports unsafe conditions.
(21) Uses good body mechanics.
(22) Maintains a positive relationship with residents, visitors, and staff.
(23) Participates in committees as requested; cooperates with, and follows safety committee, infection control committee, ergonomics committee, and quality assurance committee policies and procedures.
(24) Other duties, as assigned by supervisor.

Resident Selection Criteria/Assignment
Provides hands-on assistance at meal times. Provides hands-on assistance only to those residents with basic, uncomplicated nutrition and hydration needs. Licensed and/or certified staff members will assist residents who eat in their rooms and those with complicated feeding problems including, but not limited to, difficulty swallowing, recurrent lung aspirations, and tube or parenteral/IV feedings. The facility will base your assignment on a licensed nurse's assessment, the resident's latest care plan, and individual health needs. Because the assignment is assessment-based, it may change from day to day based on the nurse's evaluation of residents' conditions and needs.

Ethics
Honesty demands that time paid by the employer will be used profitably. If the work assigned is insufficient to occupy the time, report to the nurse in charge for additional duties. Employees must not sleep, eat, or smoke in public areas or on resident care units. Meals and break time will be assigned. Report to the nurse before leaving the unit, and again upon your return. Conserve supplies, electricity, and other commodities at all times.

This job description provides an overview of the depth, breadth, responsibilities, and requirements for the nutrition assistant. It was developed for teaching and example purposes only. It is not an exhaustive, comprehensive, or all-inclusive description of job duties, requirements, or responsibilities.

- assist residents to drink beverages
- document meal intake

A nutrition assistant *may not* physically move (transfer, pick up, lift) a resident from a wheelchair to a dining chair. He or she may not feed residents with complicated clinical conditions or difficulty swallowing, such as:

- residents with swallowing problems
- residents at risk for aspiration, a condition in which food may be accidentally inhaled into the lungs
- residents with complex feeding problems, as identified by the nurse

Responsible Employee Behavior

Responsible behavior is important for health care workers. Being responsible means you are dependable and trustworthy. Think of how you would feel if a family member was a facility resident. Residents and co-workers suffer if a member of the health care team is not responsible.

Follow rules even if you do not agree with them. Learn and profit from constructive criticism. Responsible behavior includes:

- reporting to work on time when scheduled
- keeping absences to a minimum; if you must be absent, follow facility reporting policies and give as much advance notice as possible
- keeping promises to residents and other staff members
- being dependable, so that residents and co-workers will trust you
- doing assigned tasks quickly and accurately
- demonstrating initiative; this means doing things that need to be done without being told
- cooperating with staff in all departments
- reporting safety and infection control problems
- reporting mistakes if you make them
- giving proper notice of resignation (most facilities require a minimum of two weeks' notice)

Professional appearance. You should be clean, neat, and well groomed at all times. A professional appearance makes others feel confident in you. It sends a message that you feel good about yourself and the job you do. Follow the facility dress code. Wear your identification badge at all times when on duty. Comfortable, well-fitting shoes are important. Wear shoes that are appropriate to the floor surface. Athletic shoes or sturdy shoes with closed toes provide good support. Keep your shoes clean and in good repair.

Good personal hygiene, grooming, and personal health. Staying clean is one way to maintain your personal health. You should:

- Take a bath or shower daily.
- Use deodorant or antiperspirant.
- Keep your hair clean and neat. If your hair is long, wear it up or pulled back. Style your hair to keep it out of food.
- Keep fingernails short and clean. Long fingernails injure residents. Potentially harmful germs can grow under nails. Follow facility policies for wearing acrylic nails and nail polish. Many do not allow artificial nails because they increase the risk of infection.
- Avoid fragrances and strong scents.
- Keep jewelry to a minimum when on duty. Wear simple jewelry. Elaborate settings on rings and bracelets harbor germs, and may injure a resident.
- Follow facility policies regarding tattoos and piercings.
- Wear only one pair of small, stud-type earrings. Hoops and wire earrings may be caught or pulled by a resident, causing injury.

Personal communication devices. Most facilities have policies prohibiting the use of non-work-related personal communication devices, such as cell phones and pagers. Some devices interfere with medical equipment and may jeopardize resident health and safety. Safety and care of the residents is always primary. Communication devices distract employees from this purpose. Plan to make and return phone calls during your breaks. Personal communication devices should not be worn in resident care areas. In some facilities, employees may carry electronic pagers or cellular phones set for silent alert. However, staff are not permitted to respond to calls when on duty. Remember, you are being paid to work, and stopping even briefly to make or answer calls is not part of your job description.

Organizing Your Work

Manage your time well. Practice organizing your work. Good organization reduces stress. The principles of organization will be taught by your instructor, but it is up to you to learn, practice, and master them. Report for duty at your assigned time. Get your assignment from the nurse. Learn to set priorities by doing tasks in order of importance. Anticipate needs. Have extra help and supplies ready before beginning a task. By planning and preparing in advance, the job will be much easier and you will be more efficient. Priorities sometimes change because of resident illness and other emergencies. Go with the flow and do the best you can. Avoid becoming frustrated if priorities change or must be adjusted partway through the shift.

Other Positive Qualities. While you are at work, you are on duty. You are being paid to work the whole time. Follow the rules. Report to the nurse when you go on break. Return from breaks on time. If you run out of things to do, help co-workers or perform tasks that need to be done without being told. Other positive qualities are:

- Avoid shortcuts. In health care, there is a reason for everything we do. Shortcuts can be dangerous. Do things in the manner in which you were taught.
- Perform only those procedures that you have been taught, that you have been found proficient in, and that you are permitted to do by state law and facility policies. For example, giving medication is not taught in your class. You cannot disguise a pill in food and give it to a resident. Giving pills is the nurse's responsibility.
- If you are not sure how to do something, ask the nurse or check the procedure manual.
- Inform the nurse if you will be unable to get a job done.
- Be professional at all times.
- Smile often. Greet residents, visitors, and co-workers with kindness and compassion.

CHAPTER REVIEW

Multiple Choice Questions

Select the one best answer:

1. According to the OBRA law, facilities must do all of the following *except*:
   a. provide a homelike environment.
   b. meet the residents' needs by giving them total care.
   c. maintain or improve the quality of residents' lives.
   d. promote resident independence.
2. In the long-term care facility, most of the hands-on care is provided by:
   a. registered nurses.
   b. nursing assistants.
   c. licensed practical (vocational) nurses.
   d. untrained workers.
3. The nutrition assistant's supervisor is a:
   a. dietitian.
   b. food service supervisor.
   c. nursing assistant.
   d. licensed nurse.
4. The person responsible for writing menus and making recommendations for meeting the residents' nutritional needs is the:
   a. administrator.
   b. cook.
   c. dietitian.
   d. registered nurse.
5. Responsible behavior includes:
   a. calling the facility if you are unable to come to work.
   b. coming to work when you want to.

- **c.** doing only those tasks that you want to do.
- **d.** helping the nursing assistants with resident care.

6. When at work, you should wear:
- **a.** dress clothes.
- **b.** heavy fragrances.
- **c.** acrylic nails.
- **d.** an identification badge.

7. Organize your time by:
- **a.** asking the nurse for a detailed schedule.
- **b.** avoiding conversations with residents.
- **c.** planning and preparing in advance.
- **d.** doing only what you are told to do.

8. When caring for the residents, workers should:
- **a.** follow the individual care plans.
- **b.** be as quiet as possible.
- **c.** discourage independence.
- **d.** maintain a clinical environment.

9. The nutrition assistant is qualified to:
- **a.** feed any long-term care facility resident.
- **b.** provide solid foods only.
- **c.** serve trays and assist in the dining room.
- **d.** feed stable residents with uncomplicated conditions.

10. Which of the following is *not true?*
- **a.** Taking shortcuts helps to save time.
- **b.** Being well-organized reduces worker stress.
- **c.** Workers must follow policies even if they do not agree with them.
- **d.** Personal communication devices should not be used when on duty.

UNIT 2

Resident Rights

OBJECTIVES

- Spell and define key terms.
- State the purpose of the Residents' Bill of Rights document.
- List ways in which the nutrition assistant shows respect for resident rights.
- Describe how to assist residents who are physically or mentally unable to exercise their legal rights.
- State the purpose of the Health Insurance Portability and Accountability Act.
- Define resident abuse and neglect and give one example of each.

LEGAL RIGHTS OF RESIDENTS

The long-term care facility must care for residents in a manner and in a homelike environment that:

- maintains or enhances each resident's dignity
- recognizes his or her individuality
- maintains or enhances the resident's quality of life

Residents are informed of their legal rights at the time of admission (Figure 2-1).

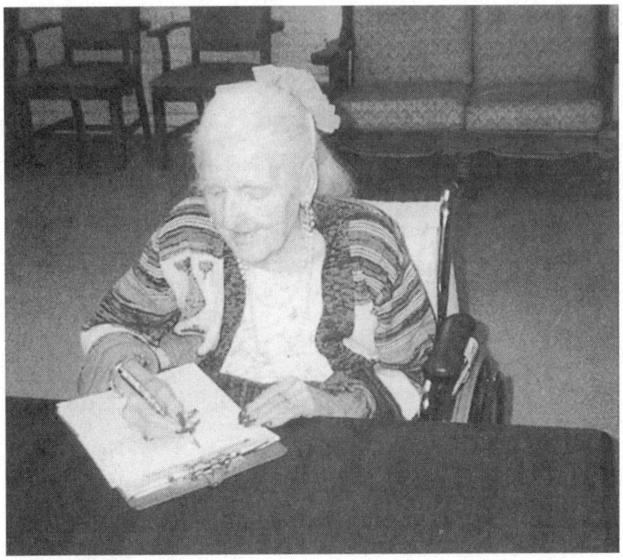

FIGURE 2-1
Residents are given a copy of the resident rights document on admission to the facility. This resident is signing an acknowledgment that she received a copy of her legal rights.

Residents' Bill of Rights

Residents in long-term care facilities have the same rights as any other citizen of the United States. The Omnibus Budget

Reconciliation Act of 1987 guarantees residents of nursing facilities certain legal rights. These rights are listed in a document called the **Residents' Bill of Rights**. The Residents' Bill of Rights is part of nursing home law. It is written in simple language. In communities with large groups of non-English-speaking persons, the bill of rights is translated into the prevalent language of the community. It applies to all residents, regardless of illness, disability, or mental status. A facility must promote the protection of rights for all residents. Residents should be able to assert their rights based on their degree of capability. Workers assist them as needed. You must be very familiar with the bill of rights. All caregivers must:

- Respect, uphold, protect, and promote the rights of each resident.
- Protect the rights of residents with mental and physical disabilities.
- Allow and assist residents to exercise their rights.

Resident rights are summarized in Box 2-1.

Confidentiality and Privacy

When people become ill, injured, old, or disabled, they may depend on others to care for them. Health care workers witness some of the most personal and intimate aspects of the human situation. We often learn things that others do not know. When you elect to work in a facility, you must abide by the standards of that organization. **Standards of care** are accepted, common health care practices. They are based on laws such as the residents' rights document, current information about health care, books, professional journals, and facility policies. Residents are guaranteed privacy and confidentiality. Workers learn personal information about residents' medical conditions. They speak with residents when giving care. Personal conversations should be held out of the hearing of others. As a result of the workers' position of trust, they learn many private details of residents' lives. Residents' right to privacy in the facility is just as important as it would be anywhere else. Employees must treat residents with dignity and respect their privacy rights. Never give information to an unauthorized person.

Assisting Residents Who Cannot Exercise Their Rights

Workers are responsible for helping residents exercise their rights if they are physically or mentally unable to do this on their own. This involves using a good deal of common sense. For example, a resident with a physical or mental impairment may not be able to cover her or his body if it is exposed. You should cover the resident. Offer to help residents who cannot do things for themselves. You may notice an unopened card on a resident's table. Offer to open and read the card to the resident. Do not open it without the resident's permission.

Give residents as much control over care and routines as possible. Always explain what you are going to do and how it will be done. Although residents may be physically unable to complete a task, they may be able to tell you how and when they want it done. Giving residents control and offering choices is an excellent way to help them exercise their rights and it promotes healthy self-esteem. It sends a message to residents that you value them as persons and respect their opinions.

Although residents are guaranteed many legal rights, they are not allowed to infringe upon the rights of others. If the rights of one resident are interfering with the rights of others, try to find a compromise. If you are unable to resolve the situation, consult the nurse.

BOX 2-1
Resident Rights

All residents in long-term care facilities have rights guaranteed to them under federal and state law. These rights include the resident's right to:

- exercise his or her rights
- a dignified existence
- self-determination
- be informed about what rights and responsibilities he or she has
- if he or she wishes, have the facility manage his or her personal funds
- choose a physician and treatment and participate in decisions and care planning
- privacy and confidentiality
- voice grievances and have the facility respond to those grievances
- examine survey results
- work or not work
- privacy in sending and receiving mail
- visit and be visited by others from outside the facility
- use a telephone in privacy
- retain and use personal possessions to the maximum extent that space and safety permit
- share a room with a spouse, if that is mutually agreeable
- self-administer medication, if the interdisciplinary care planning team determines it is safe
- refuse a transfer to or from a distinct part (skilled nursing unit) within the institution
- refuse a transfer to another room or to leave the facility unless:
  - the health and safety of the resident or others are affected
  - the facility cannot meet the resident's needs
  - the resident's condition has improved so that services are no longer required
  - the resident has not paid the bill and the facility has given the resident reasonable notice of discharge
- receive a 30-day written notice before transfer unless there are medical reasons, or the life, safety, and health of the resident or others is endangered; the resident may waive the right to the 30-day waiting period if she or he chooses
- be free from verbal, sexual, physical, and mental abuse, neglect, corporal punishment, involuntary seclusion, and misappropriation of property; the facility is responsible for caring for the resident's health, well-being, and personal possessions
- be free from any physical or chemical restraints imposed for the purposes of discipline or convenience and not required to treat medical symptoms (Rights may be restricted only to the extent necessary to protect the resident or another person from danger or harm or to protect a right of another resident, particularly those relating to privacy and confidentiality.)
- choose activities, schedules, and health care consistent with his or her interests and plan of care
- communicate, access, and interact with members of the community, persons, and services of their choosing, both inside and outside of the facility
- make choices about his or her life in the facility that are significant to the resident
- organize and participate in resident and family groups
- participate in social, religious, and community activities that do not interfere with the rights of other residents
- reside and receive services in the facility with reasonable accommodation of individual needs and preferences, except when the health or safety of the resident or others is endangered
- receive notice before the resident's room or roommate is changed

HIPAA

In 1996, Congress passed the **Health Insurance Portability and Accountability Act** (HIPAA). This law has many provisions. One portion applies to resident privacy, confidentiality, and medical records. The HIPAA policies and procedures for each facility are individualized to that facility. The concept of **protected health information** (PHI) is at the heart of the rules. The HIPAA standards list the rights of persons who are the subject of PHI. They describe the circumstances in which PHI may be disclosed. For example, PHI may be disclosed if identifying information is removed. Any hint that could lead back to the resident is considered identifiable information, including admission and discharge date, phone numbers, or pictures. The HIPAA rules:

- Restrict the use and disclosure of resident information.
- Make facilities accountable for protecting resident data and information.
- Require facilities to implement and monitor their information release policies and procedures.
- Increase residents' control over their medical records and personal information.

Under HIPAA rules, all residents have the right to:

- Know about uses and disclosure of their own PHI.
- Decide whether information can be disclosed.
- Correct inaccurate information in their records.
- Inspect their medical records.

The HIPAA regulations protect all information gathered in the care of a resident. The information may be clinical, financial, or both. All health care workers, not just physicians and nurses, must keep health information confidential. Anything workers hear, see, or create in the course of their jobs must remain confidential.

The HIPAA rules apply to verbal, paper, and electronic documentation, billing records, and clinical records. Staff working with the residents should be provided only with information that is needed to carry out their duties. Because of this, resident information is disclosed on a "need to know" basis. For example, the dietary department would need to know if the resident was on a diabetic diet. They would not need to know that the resident has an infection in an open area on the face. The nutrition assistant would probably need to know about the diabetes and the infection. Facilities must monitor how and where they use resident information. Policies must protect resident charts and records, places where resident information is discussed, faxing documents, and disclosing other personal information. For example, you may be asked to document residents' meal intake on an intake record. The record is on a clipboard that hangs on a hook on the dining room wall. For privacy, the clipboard should be covered with a piece of paper while it is being used. When residents have finished eating, the clipboard should be moved to a more secure area.

Privacy. Another important right is the residents' right to privacy in care, and when his or her body is exposed. Always knock on the door, and allow time for a response before entering a resident's room. Staff working in the room must provide complete privacy when caring for the resident. They must close the door to the room, the privacy curtain, and the window curtains. Residents must not be unnecessarily exposed. The privacy curtain and window curtains must be closed even if the door to the room is shut and no one else is in the room.

Confidentiality The law guarantees residents confidentiality in their medical care and treatment. This means that unauthorized persons may not read residents' medical records. It also means that health care workers cannot discuss personal information about residents or their conditions with others. Information about residents should only be discussed in private areas, and then only if the other person has a *need to know.* Do not discuss residents in hallways, on elevators, in the break room, or with others outside the facility. If a resident tells you something in confidence, you should not tell anyone else unless the information affects the resident's condition or medical care. For example, a resident tells you something about a private financial matter. You should not tell anyone else. However, if a resident tells you that she or he is secretly spitting out her medication, this information should be reported to the nurse. If a visitor asks you for information about a resident, refer him or her to the nurse. Residents' family members have a right to information *that the resident wants them to know.* You may tell them something about the resident's activities, such as, "She enjoyed playing BINGO this morning." For other information, refer them to the nurse. Avoid discussing residents outside the facility.

ABUSE

Abuse may be in the form of:

- willful infliction of injury
- unreasonable confinement
- intimidation
- threats
- punishment

Abuse results in physical harm, pain, or mental anguish. It can be physical, verbal, sexual, or mental. The abuser may be another resident, a family member, a staff member, or a visitor.

Types of Abuse

Abuse can take many different forms. Sometimes the abuser is not even aware that the behavior or action toward a resident is abusive. The different types of abuse are described in Table 2-1.

Recognizing signs of abuse. New bruises, pain, swelling, or other unexplained injuries to a resident may be an indication of abuse and should be reported. Other signs of possible abuse include residents responding to others with fear and anxiety. Residents who have been abused may have sudden changes in their personality or behavior. You are not

TABLE 2-1
Types of Abuse

TYPE OF ABUSE	DESCRIPTION
Physical abuse	Willful, nonaccidental injury, such as handling a resident roughly or striking, slapping, or hitting a resident
Verbal abuse	Swearing, using demeaning terms to talk to a resident, or embarrassing a resident
Mental abuse	Threatening to harm a resident, or threatening to withhold food, fluid, or care as a form of punishment
Sexual abuse	• Physical force or verbal threats are used to force a resident to perform a sexual act • Touching or fondling a resident inappropriately • Any behavior that is seductive, sexually demeaning, harassing, or reasonably interpreted as sexual by the resident

required to determine whether the changes in the resident are the result of abuse. Your responsibility is to report the observations to the nurse for further investigation.

NEGLECT

Neglect is failure to provide needed care or services. It can be deliberate or accidental. An example of neglect is forgetting to feed a resident in your assignment. As a result, the resident misses a meal. All states have laws concerning abuse and neglect of residents. Workers must report suspected or actual abuse or neglect of residents. The facility must report to law enforcement authorities and state agencies. This is a management responsibility. There are severe penalties for abusing or neglecting residents. Workers who witness abuse or neglect and do not report it may be held equally responsible for the situation. If you suspect a resident has been abused or neglected by a staff member, family, or any other individual, report this information to the nurse immediately. You are not expected to make a judgment. Report your observations only. The nurse will investigate.

Abuse and neglect may occur because a worker is feeling stressed. Residents may say things that are hurtful or upsetting. Remain calm and do not take a resident's behavior or negative remarks personally. Abuse often occurs when a worker is feeling tired, experiencing personal problems, or losing control. If you feel overwhelmed with your duties or with a resident, discuss it with the nurse or another trusted person. Arrange to take a break and compose yourself. Methods of working with residents with behavior problems will be described in Chapter 3.

CHAPTER REVIEW

Multiple Choice Questions

Select the one best answer:

1. The Residents' Bill of Rights guarantees all of the following *except:*
   a. privacy in medical treatment.
   b. confidentiality.
   c. dignified treatment.
   d. infringing on the rights of others.
2. It is acceptable to report resident information to the nurse in:
   a. a private area.
   b. the elevator.
   c. the cafeteria.
   d. the hallway.
3. A visitor asks you what is wrong with Mr. Stone, the resident in room 402. You know that Mr. Stone was recently diagnosed with pneumonia related to AIDS. Your best response is:
   a. "He has AIDS."
   b. "He has pneumonia."
   c. "I'm sorry, but I cannot give you that information."
   d. "Ask the nurse."
4. Mr. Stephens is an alert 24-year-old male resident who cannot move his arms and legs. He was admitted to the long-term care facility for rehabilitation after a serious automobile accident. Sometimes he yells at the staff. You are assigned to feed him. You should do all of the following *except:*
   a. Ask the resident what he would like to eat first.
   b. Give the resident choices as much as possible.
   c. Be as quiet as possible to avoid upsetting the resident.
   d. Introduce yourself to the resident.
5. You fed Mrs. Gianossi, a 92-year-old confused resident on Monday. Mrs. Gianossi speaks, but does not make sense. You were off on Tuesday. When you return to work on Wednesday, you are assigned to feed Mrs. Gianossi again. You notice bruises on her upper arms. You should:

a. Say nothing, as this happened on your day off.
b. Report your findings to the nurse.
c. Ask Mrs. Gianossi why she has bruises.
d. Call the police and report abuse.

6. Mr. Wolverton is a 72-year-old confused resident. You are assigned to feed him supper. He is covered with a lap blanket, but he keeps reaching underneath and tugging at it. You discover that Mr. Wolverton is soaking wet. There are brown rings of urine on his pants. There is food on his lap, and his hands are dirty. It appears as if someone did not care for this resident. This may be an example of:
   a. neglect.
   b. abuse.
   c. standards of practice.
   d. individuality.

7. Signs of abuse may include:
   a. nausea and vomiting.
   b. unexplained injuries.
   c. fever.
   d. infection.

8. Standards of care are based on all of the following *except:*
   a. laws.
   b. policies and procedures.
   c. textbooks and journals.
   d. resident and family requests.

9. When caring for residents, you should:
   a. Encourage them to eat all their food, even if they dislike it.
   b. Treat them with dignity and respect.
   c. Force them to do as much as possible.
   d. Always consult the doctor for advice.

10. The HIPAA rules:
   a. restrict medical information based on the need to know.
   b. prohibit facilities from disclosing any medical information to residents' families.
   c. require facilities to consult the doctor before releasing information.
   d. give the administrator total control over medical records and personal information.

UNIT 3

Communication and Interpersonal Skills

OBJECTIVES

- Spell and define key terms.
- List the four elements of communication.
- Define barriers to communication and give examples.
- Describe attending behavior.
- Explain why listening is an important part of communication.
- Describe how to communicate with residents.
- Identify common causes of behavior problems.
- Describe the effect of losses and unmet needs on residents' behavior.
- List the three steps in the ABC method of behavior management, and explain how this method is used to eliminate undesirable behavior.
- Describe how to communicate with residents with specific behavior problems.

COMMUNICATION

Communication involves sending and receiving messages to exchange information with others. Verbal communication is the most common method, but many forms of communication are used in health care. To be successful, you must learn and practice effective communication techniques. You will communicate with residents, families, visitors, co-workers, and managers. The messages you send and receive must be interpreted accurately. Communication is more than saying words. It is showing honest concern and caring for other people.

Factors That Influence Communication

Many factors affect the ability to communicate. Some residents have trouble seeing, hearing, or speaking. Some have language barriers or do not speak English. Some are mentally confused. Practice **empathy** when residents have difficulty communicating. Empathy is a positive quality. It involves imagining how frustrating it would be if you were standing in the resident's shoes. In this case, it involves understanding how it would feel if you could not make your needs known. Remember, empathy is understanding how the resident feels *without feeling it* for him or with him. It is connecting with, and supporting a resident when he works through difficult times. Feeling sorry for residents will not help. Try to understand residents' feelings of frustration, and help them, if possible. Your attitude is important, and affects residents' motivation. Remain positive. Listening and providing support help.

Sympathy is feeling sorry for someone because of her or his physical condition or situation. Feeling sympathetic involves *accepting others' feelings* as your own. This is a negative emotion that should be avoided. It is not healthy for you or the resident. Be patient when communicating with residents with physical and mental disabilities. Do not make assumptions about residents. For example, avoid assuming that residents who are unable to speak are confused. Residents who cannot speak often understand what is said to them. Treat all residents with dignity and respect.

ELEMENTS OF COMMUNICATION

Understanding the elements of communication will help you communicate effectively. Each message has four parts:

- **sender**—the person who originates the communication
- **message**—the information the sender wants to communicate
- **receiver**—the person for whom the communication is intended
- **feedback**—confirmation that the message was received as intended; it may be verbal or nonverbal

Verbal and Nonverbal Communication

We communicate verbally, or by the spoken word. Although your words are important, they represent only 7% of your message (Figure 3-1). The tone and pitch of your voice represents 38% of the meaning of the communication. We also use our bodies to communicate. Gestures, facial expressions, posture, and other body language represent 55% of the total communication. Your words and body language should both say the same thing.

Attending behavior shows that you are alert and interested in the message. Attending behavior involves:

- eye contact
- gestures
- posture
- body language
- physical distance from the other person
- paraphrasing

Eye contact. Good eye contact is important to communication. The eyes are powerful messengers. Even if the body is still, a great deal can be learned about how

Your Message

7% spoken word
+ 38% tone of voice
+ 55% gestures, facial expressions, posture, body language
= Total Communication

FIGURE 3-1
Your body language and tone of voice speak louder than your words.

a person is feeling or thinking by looking in the eyes. In fact, eye contact is often the most remembered part of making an impression. Your eyes communicate interest, concern, warmth, trust, feelings, and credibility. Look directly at the resident for five to seven seconds, then look away briefly. If you maintain eye contact for longer than this, the resident may become uncomfortable. Make eye contact as you finish speaking. This invites the resident to speak. In North America, eye contact is important to communication. People who do not make eye contact may be considered dishonest, insecure, or fearful. In some cultures, eye contact is avoided as a sign of respect. Be sensitive to cultural differences.

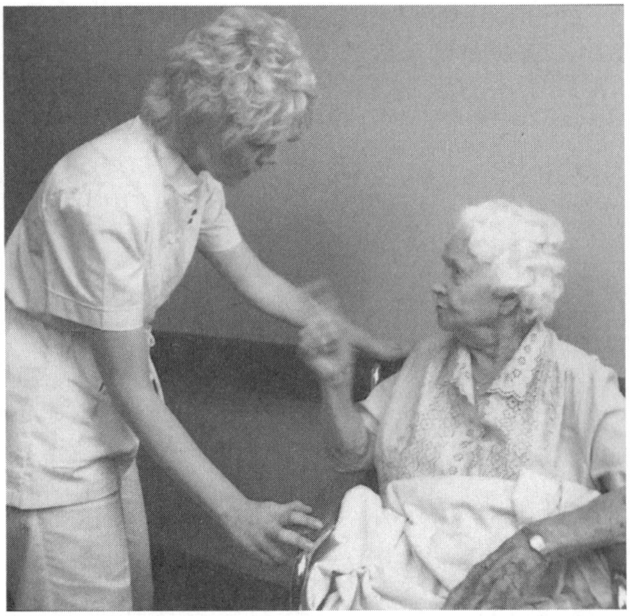

FIGURE 3-2
This resident's body language sends a message that she is very angry. The nursing assistant should maintain a neutral posture and avoid becoming defensive.

Physical distance. Physical distance is important for communication. Comfortable physical distance varies with the culture. In the United States, a comfortable physical distance is about 18 to 36 inches. If you are closer, others may be uncomfortable. If you are farther away, the receiver may be offended, or the message could be misinterpreted because the receiver cannot see or hear you.

Posture. Posture is how you hold your body when you stand, sit, or move. When you are seated, leaning forward in the chair shows that you are interested. Crossing your arms over your chest or abdomen suggests disinterest. Standing with the hands on the hips suggests anger, disgust, or impatience. Shaking a finger when you speak indicates anger (Figure 3-2). These gestures will end meaningful communication. Communication is most effective when your body is relaxed and your posture is open.

Gestures. Gestures are movements of your body or face. We gesture with our facial muscles, eyebrows, mouth, hands, and feet, or by moving about. Although we may not be aware of it, these movements send powerful messages. Use gestures and expressions only to reinforce what you say. Avoid distracting or offensive movements, such as twisting your ring, clicking your pen, playing with your hair, rolling your eyes, or moving about in your chair. These actions suggest you are bored, disinterested, or impatient. When someone else is speaking, be still. Smiling is a very effective way to communicate. A warm smile is like hanging out a welcome sign that invites people to relate to you.

Touch. Touch is a powerful means of communication. Touch can communicate a calm, caring attitude. All human beings need to be touched. Touch sends a message of compassion, caring, and acceptance. Use touch appropriate to the resident's age. Holding an adult resident's hand, or firmly resting your hand on an adult's forearm or shoulder, or patting or stroking the head of a child communicates caring. Ask the resident's permission to use touch, such as, "Would you like a hug?"

Paraphrasing. **Paraphrasing** is a means of showing that you understand what has been said. To use paraphrasing, restate your understanding of what the resident said. Listening to the message and paraphrasing provides feedback and shows that you are interested.

Barriers to Communication

A **barrier** is something that interferes with communication. It can be physical, such as trying to speak with a resident whose hearing aids are lost. Eliminate barriers whenever possible. If this is not possible, find other ways to communicate, such as writing or using adaptive communication devices (Figure 3-3). Barriers can also be mental. Mental barriers occur when you have formed a negative opinion about another person or culture. Avoid forming opinions about others based on appearances. Keep an open mind.

Other barriers may be present, such as mental confusion, speech and hearing problems, or residents who do not speak English. If you are not sure of the resident's ability to communicate, you should:

- Ask the resident's name.
- Discuss the season or weather.
- Provide orienting information, if necessary.
- Evaluate the resident's response.
- Keep your questions simple.
- Ask only one question at a time.
- Repeat or rephrase if the resident does not understand.
- Do not make fun of the resident's lack of understanding.
- Laugh with the resident, if appropriate.

GUIDELINES FOR COMMUNICATION

Use every contact with residents as an opportunity for communication. Show you value residents' worth and respect them by calling them by their preferred name. If you do not know what they prefer to be called, use Mr. or Mrs., followed by their surname. Pet names such as "honey," "dear," and "gramps" are not appropriate. Smile and speak with residents, families,

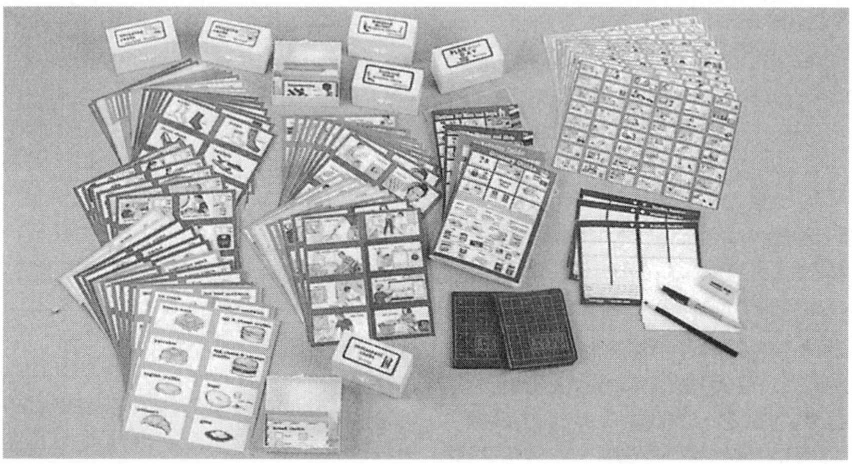

FIGURE 3-3
Pictures and similar communication devices enable residents to make their wants and needs known. The resident will point to a picture, word, or phrase to convey the message. (Picture Communication Package is provided by Sammons Preston, Inc. Reprinted with permission.)

and visitors when you pass them in the hallway. Speak with residents when giving care. Pleasant communication shows that you like and care about others.

Before beginning a conversation, set a goal. Think about what you want to accomplish and focus on the topic. Arrange the main points in logical order. Eliminate unrelated or unnecessary information that may cause confusion. Keep your message organized, clear, and complete. When residents have special communication problems, the care plan will provide information and guidance.

Guidelines for Having a Conversation

- Approach the resident in a friendly, courteous manner.
- Introduce yourself by name and title, and address the resident by his or her preferred name.
- Be polite. Use good manners.
- Choose your words carefully. Use words that are familiar to the receiver and that have only one meaning.
- Tell the resident what you plan to do.
- Allow time for the resident to ask questions and show understanding.
- If your time is limited, inform the resident how much time you have and when you will need to leave.
- Make eye contact. Sit, squat, or bend over if possible.
- Speak clearly and distinctly.
- Avoid slang or cultural terms that are unfamiliar or may be misunderstood or frightening.
- Avoid sound-alike words, such as "haul" and "hall," which are hard to understand.
- Avoid interrupting or changing the subject.
- Listen to what the resident says. Focus. Avoid distracting sights and thoughts.
- Use **open-ended questions** or make comments to encourage the resident to speak. Open-ended questions give you insight into what the resident thinks and feels. For example, say, "How does that make you feel?" Instead of saying, "Do you like the casserole?" say, "Tell me what you think about the casserole." Other ways of beginning open-ended questions are, "Tell me about. . . ," "What else. . . ," "What could. . . ," "What do you think about. . ."
- Use touch to communicate caring, if appropriate. Ask the resident's permission to use touch.
- Give facts, not opinions.
- Make messages logical, brief, and concise. Wait long enough for the resident to reply.
- Repeat the message, using exactly the same words, if necessary.
- Use nonverbal communication, such as posture, gestures, and body language, as appropriate.
- Make sure your body language matches your words and sends a positive message.
- Avoid insincere answers and false reassurance, such as "Do not worry about it," or "Everything will be all right."
- Avoid talking about your personal problems

Listening

Listening is an important part of communication. Hearing is *being aware of sound.* Listening is *an active, deliberate process* in which you focus and make an effort to hear and understand what the resident is saying. Listening can be difficult when you are distracted or have other things on your mind. Your body language may betray you by sending a message that you are not interested in what the resident is saying. Monitor your movement and expressions to avoid misunderstanding. Paraphrasing is a good technique to show that you are listening. So is silence. It shows acceptance and respect and encourages the resident to speak. If you are uncomfortable with silence, work to overcome your discomfort.

Guidelines for Listening

- Use open posture. Lean toward the resident.
- Avoid crossing your arms in front of your body or placing your hands on your hips.
- Give the resident your full attention.
- Maintain eye contact. Sit, if possible.
- Monitor the resident's body language to see if it confirms or conflicts with the verbal message.
- Be as still as possible. Monitor your own body language.
- Use open-ended questions. Encourage the resident to talk about feelings and concerns.
- Avoid passing judgment or becoming defensive if the resident expresses anger or negative feelings. Monitor your body language.
- Use touch to communicate caring, if appropriate.
- Use silence to allow the resident to think and continue the conversation.
- Show interest in the resident's activities, interests, and concerns.
- Show interest in the message. Ask questions if necessary. Paraphrase to show interest and understanding.
- Use responses such as, "I would like to hear more about that," or "Then what happened?" to show you are interested.
- Use responses, such as nodding or saying, "I understand," to show you are listening.
- Use responses such as "So you felt bad about that" to show empathy.
- Wait until the resident has finished speaking before responding.
- Request help from the nurse, if needed, to solve problems.

Guidelines for Communicating with Residents with Disabilities

In addition to the general guidelines for communication and listening, use the following methods when communicating with persons with disabilities:

- Avoid referring to the resident as a condition, such as "the stroke in 221." Say instead, "Mrs. Smith in 221." Emphasize the person over the condition. For example, do not say, "the diabetic." Instead use, "the person with diabetes."
- Use common sense. Speak the same way you would with anyone else. People with disabilities do not want to be treated differently.
- Do not assume that someone is *not disabled* or pretending because the disability is not visible. Some medical conditions are severely disabling, but the person may not appear disabled.
- Never assume that the resident can or cannot do something. Assuming is offensive. Always ask. Before helping a person with a disability, ask if you can help. It is all right to offer to help, but unless the resident is struggling, do not assume that the person needs help without asking.
- It is all right to ask residents about their disabilities. Many residents are comfortable, and will talk about them, but it is also all right if they do not want to talk about it.

- Always stress the ability and not the disability.
- Avoid making assumptions about individuals with mobility aids. They are not always sick.
- Residents in wheelchairs do not like to be treated as if they are mentally impaired! Most have no mental problem. Talk to the person in the wheelchair, not a companion.
- When talking to a resident in a wheelchair, position yourself at eye level.
- Use good manners if you walk in front of a resident in a wheelchair by excusing yourself.
- Avoid standing in front of a person in a wheelchair, which blocks the resident's view.
- The wheelchair is an extension of the disabled person's body. Leaning or hanging on the chair is an invasion of the resident's personal space.
- Words such as "see," "hear," "run," and "walk" can be used when speaking with people with disabilities.
- Choose words that are positive and nonjudgmental.
- Avoid words like "cripple," "gimp," "spastic," "retard." These are demeaning and promote negative perceptions of persons with disabilities.
- People with disabilities like to laugh and have fun. Do not leave them out!
- Canine companions, such as seeing eye dogs or hearing ear dogs, are on duty. Do not feed them or pet them without the owner's permission.
- If you do not understand what the resident says, ask him or her to repeat it.
- Accept responsibility for being unable to understand a message. The resident is doing his or her best and is probably more frustrated than you are. Do not discourage or blame the resident for the breakdown in communication. Consult the nurse.

Communicating with Residents with Vision Loss

Vision loss can range from problems that can be corrected with glasses to complete blindness. Some people are legally blind, but still have limited vision. Avoid assuming that residents wearing glasses can see. Some residents wear glasses but are severely impaired. People with vision problems are like residents with other disabilities. They may have a loss in one area of their life, but they have developed other areas. Many are self-sufficient, but may need environmental adaptations. Do not rearrange furniture, equipment, supplies, or personal items without informing the resident. People with visual impairments memorize the location of items. Moving things could result in accidents, injuries, or frustration because the resident is unable to find a needed item. When you would like the resident to do something, provide detailed, step-by-step directions.

Communicating with Residents with Hearing Loss

Hearing loss can mean that a resident has difficulty hearing or is completely deaf. Hearing loss has many causes. Treatment is determined by the cause. Some residents will benefit from hearing aids or ear surgery. However, others have uncorrected hearing loss. The care plan will provide special instructions for communicating with the resident. Placing a stethoscope into the resident's ears, then speaking into the bell or diaphragm works for some. Some residents use sign language, which combines hand signals and facial expressions. Others read lips. Some use reading and writing to communicate. Special telephone, television, computer communication systems, and amplifiers are available for people with hearing loss. Residents with hearing loss can often function independently, but may need environmental adaptations.

Communicating with Residents Who Have Problems with Language and Understanding

Some residents have conditions affecting their ability to speak or understand what is spoken to them. They may be able to understand some things, but not others. Try to communicate with them as you would other residents. Do not make the mistake of being silent. Silence may be received as a negative message by the resident. You must assume that the resident understands you. Use short, simple words and phrases. Pronounce them clearly and slowly. Focus on one topic and use short sentences. The resident may be able to speak, but may not make sense. Some residents have certain words or phrases that have meaning to them, but not to you. Listen and try to understand what they are saying. Be empathetic and do not show frustration. If you learn what they are saying, inform the nurse. Some residents cannot speak, but understand what is said to them. Do not assume that residents with speech problems are confused. Test the resident's ability to answer yes or no questions, or to follow simple directions to determine understanding.

Communicating with Residents Who Have Problems Speaking

Some diseases and injuries leave residents unable to speak. They may be able to make noise, but not form words. However, they often understand what you are saying. Do not make the mistake of thinking a resident is confused because of the speech problem. With therapy, some residents will regain their speech. Some use other methods of communication. The resident may be able to communicate by using gestures, writing, or adaptive communication devices. Use questions that can be answered with yes or no answers. Tell the resident to nod his or her head in response. If the resident is unable to nod the head, tell him or her to blink the eyes once for yes and twice for no. Accept responsibility for being unable to understand a message. Consult the nurse, if necessary.

Communicating with Residents Who Have Cognitive Impairment

Good communication skills are necessary when caring for residents with cognitive impairment (confusion). Reduce distractions or move to an area that is free from disruptions. These residents have lost the ability to screen out distractions and noises from the television, radio, or other conversations. Other suggestions are:

- Monitor your body language. Make sure it sends the proper message and does not communicate impatience or anger.
- Call the resident by name and tell her or him who you are.
- Begin your conversation with orienting information.
- Make eye contact and be sure you have the resident's attention before beginning to speak.
- Sit at the resident's eye level when speaking, whenever possible.
- Begin your conversation socially to win the resident's trust. One way of doing this is by sitting and visiting.

- After the resident is relaxed, explain what you are going to do.
- If the resident ignores you, wait a minute and try again. Gently touch the resident's arm to get her or his attention. However, avoid startling the resident.
- Speak slowly and clearly, using short, simple sentences.
- Ask questions that require a yes or no answer.
- Use concrete terms and familiar words.
- Keep your tone of voice low, and speak in a calm, warm, pleasant manner.

You may have trouble understanding what the resident tells you. Listen actively and carefully. If you do not understand, apologize and ask the resident to repeat. Try to focus on a word or phrase that you understand. Repeat what you do understand and help the resident clarify it. Respond to the resident's emotion. For example, say, "You sound very angry." Remain calm and patient. If the resident repeats certain words, ask staff and family members if they know the meaning. Sometimes people with cognitive impairment talk by using code words that close friends and family understand.

Residents with cognitive impairment lose the ability to reason. Try these approaches:

- Avoid arguing, which makes the situation worse.
- Do not tell the resident what she or he can and cannot do. Instead, use distraction.
- The resident may say, "I'm going home to cook dinner for my children." You know the children are grown and live in another state. Instead of arguing with the resident, ask what she likes to cook. Talk to her about cooking. Then distract her by asking her to sit with you and look at a cooking magazine. *She is looking for a state of mind, not a location.* Discussing cooking restores the state of mind she is seeking.
- Avoid asking the resident questions that require a good memory. People with dementia recognize they have memory loss and may be humiliated and frustrated when they can't remember.
- Never talk about confused residents in front of them. Never make fun of a resident. We do not know what they understand, and their understanding changes from one moment to the next.

DEVELOPING RELATIONSHIPS

Using good communication and interpersonal skills will help you form positive relationships. Positive qualities that will help you form relationships are:

- patience—being calm and even-tempered
- courtesy—using good manners and showing respect and consideration for others
- tact—being considerate, polite, and thoughtful; having a sense of what to say or do to form and maintain good relationships and avoid offense
- empathy—the ability to understand another's point of view and share in another's feelings or emotions

Guidelines for Developing Relationships

In addition to the guidelines for communication and listening, use the following guidelines for developing relationships with residents and others:

- Make an effort to develop positive relationships with residents and others.
- If you see a need, offer to help.
- Show initiative, be a self-starter.
- Avoid insincere comments, such as, "I know how you feel."
- Communicate with residents when caring for them. If other staff are present, do not speak to them exclusively. *Always include the resident in conversation.*
- Show respect.
- Always give residents choices; allow them to have as much control as possible.
- Be supportive when a resident discusses a problem.

BEHAVIOR PROBLEMS

Behavior problems often have medical, social, or emotional causes. These problems create a great deal of stress for residents. Some behavior problems are related to a decline in intellectual functioning called **cognitive impairment**. Problem behaviors may cause danger to the resident, staff, and others. Some behaviors may be annoying or distressing, but are harmless. Behavior problems to report are listed in Box 3-1. Caring for residents with behavior problems requires using patience, common sense, good communication skills, and empathy.

Unmet Needs

Many people develop behavior problems in response to stress, loss, and unmet needs that exceed their coping ability. Residents with behavior problems who are alert are probably responding to an unmet psychosocial need, such as feelings of lack of control over their body, their situation, or the environment. You may be able to assist this resident by:

- getting to know the resident and respecting her or his uniqueness as a person
- giving the resident control and choices, which shows respect

BOX 3-1
Behavior Observations to Make and Report

Always report abnormal behavior to the nurse, even if you believe the behavior is "normal for the resident."

Who? Does the behavior involve another person or specific types of people? How are these individuals alike?

What? Describe the behavior. What were the circumstances in which the behavior occurred?

Where? Did the behavior occur in one specific location?

When? What is the time of day? Does the behavior occur at predictable times or in predictable situations, such as during bathing? When the resident is tired, when the resident awakens, and so on?

What were the environmental conditions? Was it light, dark, hot, cold, noisy, quiet?

How do others respond to the resident's behavior? Is there anyone who is never approached by the resident? If so, how does he or she manage or prevent the behavior?

Is there a pattern or clues to the behavior? Can you identify clues or signals that the behavior is about to begin?

- promoting and rewarding independence, decision making, and positive behavior

If you identify the resident's unmet needs, inform the nurse. This will help in developing a care plan to meet the needs and eliminate the behavior problems.

Residents who are mentally confused may act out in response to:

- fear
- loneliness
- boredom
- too much or too little stimulation in the environment
- unmet physical needs

Certain behaviors may be the only way residents have to express themselves. For example, a confused resident screams frequently. This is challenging because there are so many potential reasons for the screaming. She may be hungry or thirsty, in pain, hot, cold, scared, lonely, or bored. She may need to use the bathroom, but is unable to tell you. She may be agitated and reacting to too much noise and confusion. The only way to find out is by using common sense and experimenting with different approaches. Offer her a drink or something to eat. Walk with her to the bathroom, or ask a nursing assistant to take her. Sit quietly and hold her hand. Rubbing lotion on the resident's hands and arms often has a calming effect. Inform the nurse if you find an approach that calms the resident.

The meaning of behavior problems. All behavior has a meaning; it just might not be apparent to you. A resident may not even realize that he or she is behaving badly. This is often true if the resident is from a different culture. Behavior that is acceptable in one culture may be considered abnormal by people from other cultures. Also, behavior patterns develop throughout a person's lifetime.

Residents react to losses using coping and defense mechanisms they have learned over their lifetime. Use good communication and listening skills. Understand that residents are responding to stress when they use coping mechanisms. Do not take angry outbursts or other behavior personally. Although the resident may say she is angry with you, this is probably untrue. She is angry because of her situation. Monitor how the resident responds to you, then adjust your approach. Practice empathy and try to understand what is happening. Tell the resident, "I see you are upset." Encourage her to talk about it. Be a good listener.

THE ABCs OF BEHAVIOR MANAGEMENT

An effective technique of behavior management is the ABC plan (Table 3-1). This plan is useful for both alert and confused residents. The theory for this technique is that if the **antecedent** or **consequences** are eliminated or modified, the behavior will change or cease. The antecedent is the event that causes or triggers a behavior. The consequences are the outcome of the behavior.

TABLE 3-1
The ABCs of Behavior Management

IDENTIFY THE ABCS	DEFINITION
A = Antecedent	The cause or trigger of the behavior
B = Behavior	The behavior itself
C = Consequences	The consequences, effects, or results of the behavior

The Three Steps of Behavior Management

There are three steps in the ABC method of behavior management:

- Step 1—Attempt to determine the cause (trigger or antecedent) of the behavior. Does it occur in certain environmental conditions, at a certain time of day, or during a certain activity? Does the presence or absence of other persons trigger the behavior?
- Step 2—Eliminate the cause of the behavior. If the cause can be identified and eliminated, the behavior will cease or change.
- Step 3—Examine the consequences of the behavior. They may also have to be eliminated or changed in order to change the behavior. Modifying the consequences of behavior requires practice. For example, a confused resident yells and cries. You discover that if you sit and hold the resident's hand, the behavior stops. Sitting and holding a hand rewards the behavior. To modify the consequences, sit and hold the resident's hand *before* the yelling and crying starts. Pay regular attention to the resident. In this case, modifying the consequences changes the behavior. However, if the resident's behavior has been rewarded for a long time, it will not change immediately. All team members will have to practice the new approach consistently before results are apparent.

If a resident displays a behavior problem, the care plan likely deals with it. The plan is based on the resident's strengths and needs. It will describe how to reduce the behavior problem. Sometimes this is done by ignoring the behavior, if this can safely be done. Never punish the resident. The goal is to show the resident a more positive way of directing energy. For the plan to be effective, resident care must be **consistent**. All staff must follow the care plan. The plan may call for you to modify your own behavior in response to the resident's behavior. Residents tend to repeat behavior that is rewarded. Verbal praise, positive feedback, and other signs of approval are rewards. Nonverbal reinforcement such as a hug, smile, or pat on the back may also be used. Snacks and privileges are sometimes used as rewards.

Guidelines for Assisting Residents with Behavior Problems

- If the care plan calls for you to respond when a resident displays a certain behavior, begin as soon as the behavior starts. Do not wait for the resident to lose control.
- Maintain control of your own responses and reactions.
- Attempt to learn the cause of the behavior, and communicate this information to the nurse.
- Remove the irritant (cause of the behavior), if known.
- Protect the safety of the resident and others.
- Use good communication and listening skills.
- Practice empathy.
- Monitor the resident's response to your approaches. Adjust your approach if necessary.
- Discuss family, friends, or other pleasant information with residents. This provides a source of strength, comfort, and support.
- Make certain the resident's physical needs are met.
- Give alert residents as much control as possible. Offer choices whenever possible. Allow them to direct their own care.
- Be happy. Smile to communicate caring. Make sure your body language does not send a negative message. Positive behavior is contagious.

Complaining, demanding behavior. Listening to resident complaints requires a great deal of tact. Sometimes resident complaints are justified, but at times they are not. Listen to what the resident says. Report the information to the nurse objectively. If the complaint is something simple that you can correct, do so immediately.

Guidelines for Assisting the Resident with Complaining/Demanding Behavior

- Reassure the resident that you understand the complaint or problem and will report it to the appropriate person.
- Use good listening skills and support the resident.
- If the complaints are about care given by others, remain neutral. Never criticize other workers. If complaints are about your care, listen, but do not argue or become defensive.
- Attempt to determine the cause of unjustified complaints and correct it, if possible.
- Offer the resident choices and give the resident as much control over daily routines as possible.
- Show respect for the resident as a person, and demonstrate that you value her or his opinion.

Yelling and screaming. Yelling and screaming may be the only way some residents can communicate or express displeasure. Most screaming behavior is seen in confused residents, but occasionally alert residents also yell and scream. Dealing with this type of behavior is usually done by trial and error.

Guidelines for Assisting the Resident Who is Yelling/Calling Out

- Look for the cause of the behavior. If you can identify it, correct it.
- If the resident is alert, ask what the problem is. Use active listening skills and provide comfort.
- Realize that it is socially acceptable in some cultures to scream with pain and grief.
- Offer the resident something to eat or drink.
- Monitor body language to see if the resident grimaces or shows other signs of pain.
- Try to distract the resident. Redirect the resident with a positive activity, such as a walk or looking at a picture album.
- Eliminate or reduce environmental stimulation. Try moving the resident to a quiet area.
- Determine if the resident needs to use the bathroom. Screaming may be caused by the discomfort of a full bladder.

Physical or verbal aggression. Physical aggression is hitting, scratching, kicking, biting, or fighting. This is called **combative behavior**. Verbal aggression is arguing, accusing, threatening, or swearing.

Guidelines for Assisting the Aggressive Resident

- Attempt to identify the cause of the behavior and eliminate it, if possible.
- Respect the resident's need for personal space.
- Take physical threats seriously and keep your distance.
- Watch the resident's eyes. They will usually focus on the part of the body to be attacked.
- Remain calm.
- Speak in a soft, low, calm, firm voice.
- Do not make the resident feel trapped or cornered. Do not turn your back on the resident.

- Do not respond with anger or hostility. Monitor your body language and tone of voice.
- Avoid touching the resident, as this may cause further agitation.
- Show that you are interested in what the resident is saying.
- Emphasize with the resident and acknowledge that you understand he or she is upset.
- Reassure the resident.
- Praise efforts at self-control.
- Do not argue or try to reason with the resident.
- Make sure your body language is not threatening.
- If aggressive behavior occurs in a public area, move the resident if it is safe to do so. If not, move others out of the way.
- Distract or move the resident, if possible.
- Call for assistance from others, if necessary.

CHAPTER REVIEW

Multiple Choice Questions

Select the one best answer:

1. Empathy means:
   a. understanding how the resident feels.
   b. feeling sorry for the resident.
   c. understanding emotional needs.
   d. solving problems for the resident.
2. The sender is the person who:
   a. gets the message.
   b. initiates a communication.
   c. interprets the message.
   d. relays communication to another person.
3. Feedback is:
   a. your interpretation of your assignment.
   b. your interpretation of what the resident said.
   c. confirmation a message was received as intended.
   d. confirmation that you heard something.
4. Which of the following are components of attending behavior?
   a. Eye contact and gestures.
   b. Thinking and feeling.
   c. Crossing your arms and legs.
   d. Tone of voice and moving your hands.
5. Comfortable personal space in the United States is:
   a. 8 inches to 10 inches.
   b. 18 inches to 36 inches.
   c. 28 inches to 42 inches.
   d. 48 inches to 64 inches.
6. Paraphrasing is:
   a. repeating what the speaker says word for word.
   b. interpreting the message for another person.
   c. using sign language for a deaf resident.
   d. restating a message in clear, simple terms.
7. Something that interferes with communication is a:
   a. gesture.
   b. barrier.
   c. suggestion.
   d. symptom.
8. Thinking about what you want to accomplish in a conversation and focusing on a topic is an example of using:
   a. goal-oriented communication.
   b. paraphrasing.
   c. empathy.
   d. feedback communication.
9. When caring for residents with problems with speech or understanding, you should:
   a. Explain the care you will be giving in medical terms.
   b. Choose short, simple words and use short sentences.

c. Use sign language that the resident understands.
d. Avoid explaining anything because the resident will not understand.

10. According to the ABC method of behavior management:
a. "A" is an abbreviation for anger.
b. "A" is an abbreviation for anxiety.
c. "B" is an abbreviation for behavior.
d. "C" is an abbreviation for control.

11. Behavior problems are often caused by:
a. anger with the staff.
b. disliking the food.
c. stress and unmet needs.
d. desire to leave the facility.

12. A cognitively impaired resident displays a behavior problem. She yells and screams loudly. A good first step in managing this behavior is:
a. telling the resident to stop disturbing others.
b. asking a nursing assistant what to do.
c. isolating the resident.
d. attempting to learn the cause of the behavior.

13. When an alert resident displays a behavior problem, it is often in response to:
a. unmet psychosocial needs.
b. cognitive impairment.
c. unmet physical needs.
d. anger at the nutrition assistant.

14. When caring for residents with behavior problems:
a. Politely ask the resident not to disturb others.
b. Try to reason with the resident.
c. Implement the behavior care plan immediately.
d. Remove the resident from the area.

15. Common causes of agitation in cognitively impaired residents include:
a. noise and confusion in the environment.
b. anger at the staff.
c. disliking the other residents.
d. abuse and neglect.

UNIT 4

Preventing the Spread of Infection

OBJECTIVES

- Spell and define key terms.
- List three ways that infection is spread.
- Describe things you can do to prevent the spread of infection.
- Demonstrate the correct handwashing procedure.
- Demonstrate how to apply and remove gloves.
- Describe how bloodborne pathogens are spread and list measures to take to prevent the spread of bloodborne pathogens to yourself and others.
- Define standard precautions and describe why, how, and when they are used.

INFECTION

Infection is a state of illness caused by foreign organisms in the body. Preventing the spread of infection is an important responsibility. **Infection control** involves practices that prevent the spread of infection. Infection control protects you and your family members, residents and their family members, other staff members, and visitors to the health care facility.

Microorganisms are also called **microbes**. They are living organisms that are present everywhere in the environment. We cannot see them with the eye. Some are harmless and do not cause disease. **Normal flora** are healthy microbes that are helpful to the function of the body. For example, the normal flora in the digestive tract help break down food and turn it into waste products. However, when these organisms enter an area of the body where they do not belong, they may cause disease.

Pathogens are microbes that cause disease. **Bacteria** are microorganisms that can be eliminated with **antibiotics. Viruses** are tiny pathogens that cause many diseases and cannot be eliminated by antibiotics. However, vaccines can prevent many viruses. We can destroy many pathogens in the environment by a process known as **disinfection**. This involves scrubbing or soaking an item with a chemical or cleaning agent. The item is rinsed to remove all traces of the chemical. **Sterilization** eliminates all microbes and is done by using heat, gas, or chemicals.

SPREAD OF INFECTION

Infection is spread by many methods. The most common are:

- **direct contact**—touching an infected person, such as when shaking hands.
- **indirect contact**—touching environmental surfaces and objects such as soiled linen, supplies, equipment, countertops, door knobs, or faucets that have unseen pathogens on them.
- **airborne** route—pathogens enter the air in respiratory secretions. A cough or sneeze expels them into the air. The pathogens are lightweight, and are picked up in air currents, by the ventilation system, in dust, or on moisture particles in the air. They may travel long distances.
- **droplet** method—droplets are also respiratory secretions. Pathogens spread by droplets are larger and heavier than those spread by the airborne method. Because of their size and weight, they usually do not spread beyond 3 feet from the infected person.
- **common vehicle**—items that we ingest, such as food, water, or medications, may contain pathogens.
- **vectors**—insects, rodents, and small animals that carry pathogens.

Pathogens spread by direct and indirect contact usually enter your body by way of your hands. Pathogens commonly enter the body through:

- breaks in the skin
- contact with mucous membranes of the eyes, nose, mouth, and respiratory tract
- inhalation from the air

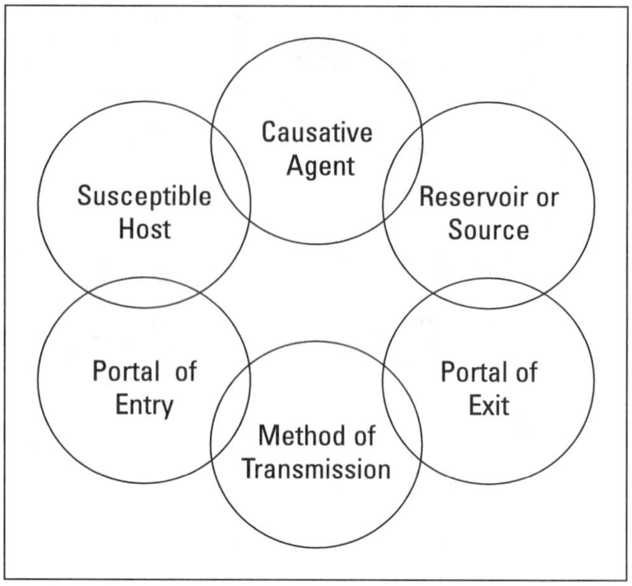

FIGURE 4-1
The chain of infection demonstrates the six factors that must come together in order to contract an infection. Your objective is to use good infection control practices to keep them apart. If one link of the chain is broken or missing, infection cannot develop.

The Chain of Infection

The **chain of infection** (Figure 4-1) describes six factors necessary for an infection to develop.

- The **source** represents the agent that causes disease.
- The **reservoir** is the place where the pathogens live and grow. They thrive in warm, moist, dark places.
- The **portal of entry** is the place where microbes enter the body.
- The **portal of exit** is how the pathogens leave the body, such as in urine, stool, blood, body fluids, secretions, excretions, or droplets.
- The **mode of transmission** is the method by which the disease is spread.
- The **susceptible host** is the person who can get an infection. People who are young, very old, have

certain diseases, or use poor infection control practices are very susceptible.

If any part of the chain of infection is broken, the disease will not spread. Infection control practices are used to break the links in the chain.

Guidelines for Reducing the Spread of Infection

- Wash your hands often.
- Keep the work area neat, tidy, and sanitary.
- Clean equipment after each use.
- Handle and dispose of soiled material properly.
- Practice good personal hygiene.
- Handle food properly.
- Handle clean and soiled items correctly.
- Keep clean and soiled items separate.
- Perform procedures in the way that you were taught without taking shortcuts.

Many infections are spread by the hands. Because of this, special attention must be given to hand hygiene. Keep the skin on your hands in good condition. Outside the facility, wear gloves when performing tasks such as gardening or washing dishes. Use hand lotion to prevent cracking, drying, and irritation. Many facilities do not permit workers to wear artificial fingernails. Keep natural nailtips less than ¼-inch long. Long and artificial nails hold microbes and increase the risk of infection. They are difficult to clean and may tear gloves. Chipped nail polish also hides germs. Wear only simple rings, such as a plain wedding band. Rings with many stones and elaborate settings can hide pathogens and are difficult to clean. The stones and settings on rings may also tear gloves. Microbes may also hide under the rings.

Separation of Clean and Soiled Items and Equipment

To prevent infection, clean and soiled items must be kept separate. Clean items are either new, wrapped articles or reusable articles that have been washed or cleaned by staff. Soiled items are things used by a resident or brought into a resident's room. They are considered soiled even if they were not used to care for the resident. They must be cleaned or disinfected after they are removed from the room. They cannot be used in the care of another resident.

Guidelines for Separating Clean and Soiled

- Keep the food cart and clean linen cart separated from the soiled linen hamper and housekeeping cart by at least one room's width. The food cart and clean linen cart are clean items. The linen hamper and housekeeping cart are contaminated items.
- Remove the housekeeping cart(s) from the hallway when food trays are being served. Many facilities also remove soiled linen hampers at mealtime.
- Many facilities have pets. They should not enter areas where food is being prepared or served. If you touch a pet, wash your hands.
- Store clean and soiled items in the designated area.
- Bring only needed supplies into the resident's room.
- Avoid carrying trash or other contaminated items next to your clothing.
- Dispose of trash contaminated with blood or body fluid according to facility policy in covered containers in a special storage area.
- Wear gloves and other protective equipment if contact with blood,

body fluid, mucous membranes, secretions, or excretions is likely.

- Wear gloves if you have nonintact (cut, chapped, or cracked) skin on your hands, or if you must touch an area of the resident's body that is not intact.
- Use liquid soap for handwashing whenever possible.
- If gloves are needed, use them for the care of one resident only, then discard.
- Gloves are contaminated after resident contact. Do not touch clean supplies, linen, equipment, or environmental surfaces with used gloves. If necessary, remove one glove and use your ungloved hand to touch other items or surfaces. You may place a clean paper towel under one glove and contact surfaces with the towel.
- Dispose of used gloves according to facility policy. They are usually discarded in covered or closed containers, not open wastebaskets.
- Lab specimens are *never* stored in the refrigerator with food or beverages.
- Follow your assignment and facility cleaning schedule. Special cleaners are used for permanent items. The friction created by wiping is important to remove microbes. Make sure supplies are completely dry before storing them.
- Resident water pitchers should be covered. Water pitchers and cups in resident rooms should be marked so they are not accidentally mixed up.
- Cover food and beverages when you carry them in the hallway.
- Store resident snacks and food items in covered containers or sealed packages, according to facility policy. Date them when they are stored.
- Leave trays on the food cart until you are ready to feed residents to maintain temperature.
- Close the door to the food cart as soon as you remove a tray to maintain food temperature and prevent contamination.
- Do not return a used tray to the food cart until after all clean trays have been served.
- Plan and organize your time so you are available to pass trays as soon as the cart is delivered. Food must be served promptly to maintain temperature.
- Never serve perishable food or beverages left at room temperature for two hours or more without refrigeration. Discard the items and obtain fresh ones.
- Refrigerate perishable leftovers as soon as possible. Never let them sit for more than one hour if the cooked temperature was more than 90 degrees F. All other leftover items must be refrigerated within two hours or discarded.
- Store perishable items correctly in the refrigerator. Follow facility policies.
- Never use food products or supplement items after the expiration date.
- Never serve food items if packages are damaged.
- Monitor residents for hoarding or improperly storing food.
- Monitor residents for unsafe behavior, such as taking food and utensils off the plates of other residents.

CLEANING YOUR HANDS

Handwashing is the most important method of preventing the spread of infection. You can pick up microbes on your hands and introduce them to your own body. You can also transfer the microbes on your hands to residents. If your hands touch a clean object, the microbes may be transferred there. You can pick up microbes from a contaminated surface or item. The purpose of handwashing is to clean the hands and prevent microorganisms from spreading. Handwashing should take a minimum of 15 seconds. If your hands are visibly soiled, you will need to take longer. The longer the handwashing, the more microbes are eliminated. The most important part of the handwashing procedure is the friction caused by rubbing your hands together. The friction removes the microbes from your hands.

Guidelines for Times When Handwashing Should Be Done

- when coming on duty
- after picking up anything from the floor
- before applying and after removing gloves
- before and after feeding each resident (or assisting with a beverage)
- before passing fresh drinking water
- after picking up soiled food trays
- after personal use of the toilet
- after you cough or sneeze, or use a tissue to blow your nose
- before and after applying lip balm
- before and after manipulating contact lenses
- before and after eating, drinking, or smoking
- before handling a resident's food and drink
- after contact with anything considered soiled or contaminated
- before handling any supply considered clean
- immediately if your hands contact blood, moist body fluid except sweat, mucous membranes, nonintact skin, secretions, or excretions even if gloves were worn during the contact
- whenever your hands are visibly soiled
- before treating a cut or break on your own skin
- after handling uncooked foods, particularly raw meat, poultry, or fish
- after touching an animal (especially a reptile)
- after handling trash or garbage
- after touching anything that many people have handled
- after touching equipment or environmental surfaces that might be contaminated (such as when moving a soiled linen hamper or housekeeping cart)
- any time your gloves become torn
- before you go on break and at the end of your shift before you leave the facility

Rules for Handwashing

- Turn the faucets on and off with a clean, dry paper towel.
- Quickly rinsing your hands with water, then drying them with a towel does not remove germs. Oils on your skin must be washed away, along with attached germs. Use warm water, soap, and friction. Spend at least 15 seconds to wash the germs away.
- Avoid leaning against the sink. The inside of the sink and the faucet handles are contaminated. The outside of the sink may contaminate your clothing.
- Avoid splashing your clothing when washing your hands.
- Keep your fingertips pointed down during the handwashing procedure.

- Bar soap can hold microorganisms on its surface. Use liquid soap whenever possible.
- Wash under and around your rings.
- Wash under and around your fingernails.
- Never wash your gloved hands. Handwashing damages the gloves so they will not protect you. Remove gloves, wash your hands, then reapply a clean pair of gloves.

Procedure 1—Handwashing

1. Turn on warm water using a paper towel.
2. Wet your hands. Keep your fingertips pointed down.
3. Apply soap from the dispenser.
4. Rub your hands together vigorously to create a lather. Then rub your hands in a circular motion for 15 seconds. Rub all surfaces of the hands. Pay particular attention to the area between your fingers. Keep your fingertips pointed down (Figure 4-2).
5. Rub your fingernails against the palm of the opposite hand. Clean your nails with a brush or an orange stick if they are soiled.
6. Rinse your hands from the wrist to the fingertips. Keep the fingers pointed down.
7. Dry your hands with a paper towel.
8. Use a clean, dry paper towel to turn off the faucet (Figure 4-3). Do not touch the faucet handle with your hands.
9. Discard the paper towel.

Waterless Hand Cleaners

Many facilities provide dispensers containing waterless hand cleaners. These hand cleaners contain an alcohol-based gel, lotion, or foam that is dispensed in small portions. Alcohol-based products are often less irritating to the hands than

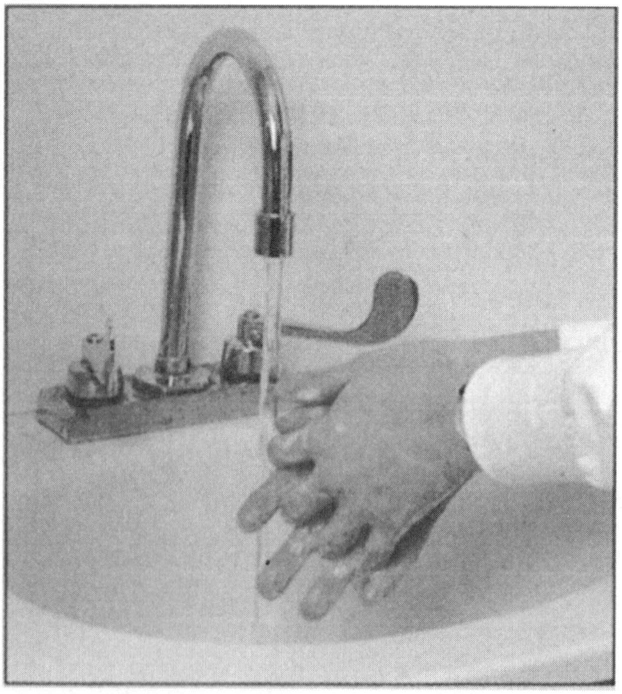

FIGURE 4-2
Friction is important to remove germs. Rub all surfaces well for at least 15 seconds.

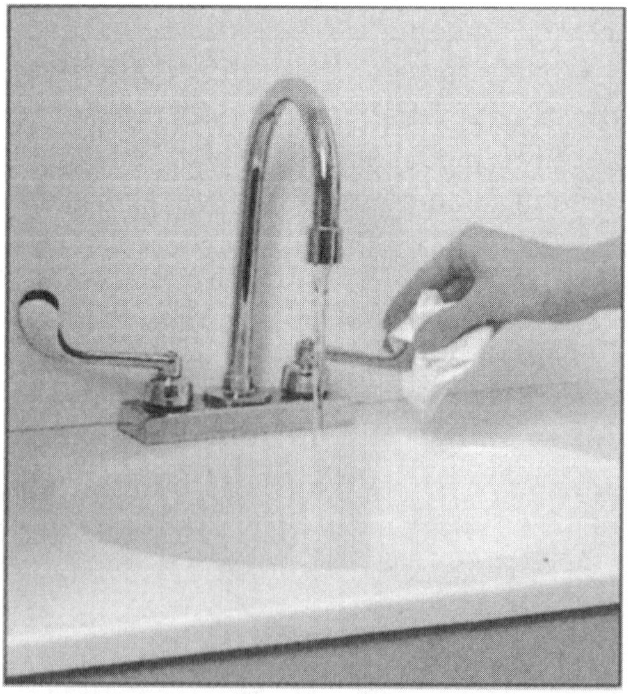

FIGURE 4-3
The faucets hold germs that were left by dirty hands. Always use a towel to turn the faucet off.

washing repeatedly with soap. Most alcohol solutions contain moisturizers that prevent drying of the skin. In addition, paper towels are not necessary when alcohol products are used. Paper towels contain wood fibers that can be very irritating to sensitive skin.

Each facility has directions for using these products and policies and procedures for when the waterless hand cleaners may be used. Waterless hand cleaner may be safely used instead of handwashing during routine resident care. However, washing at the sink should be done any time the hands are visibly soiled. To use the waterless cleaning product, dispense the proper amount into the palm of your hand. Rub the product into the hands until it dries, making sure to rub all areas and surfaces, including the nail beds and between the fingers. This should take at least 15 seconds. Become familiar with the products used by your facility and their applications. They are effective in reducing infection and eliminating pathogens from the hands.

USING STANDARD PRECAUTIONS

Health care workers must take measures to prevent the spread of infection to themselves and others. These measures are called **standard precautions** (Figure 4-4). We cannot tell whether someone has a disease or infection by appearance. Because of this, standard precautions are used in the care of all residents, regardless of their disease or diagnosis. Standard precautions protect workers against many diseases.

Standard precautions involve the use of **personal protective equipment (PPE)**

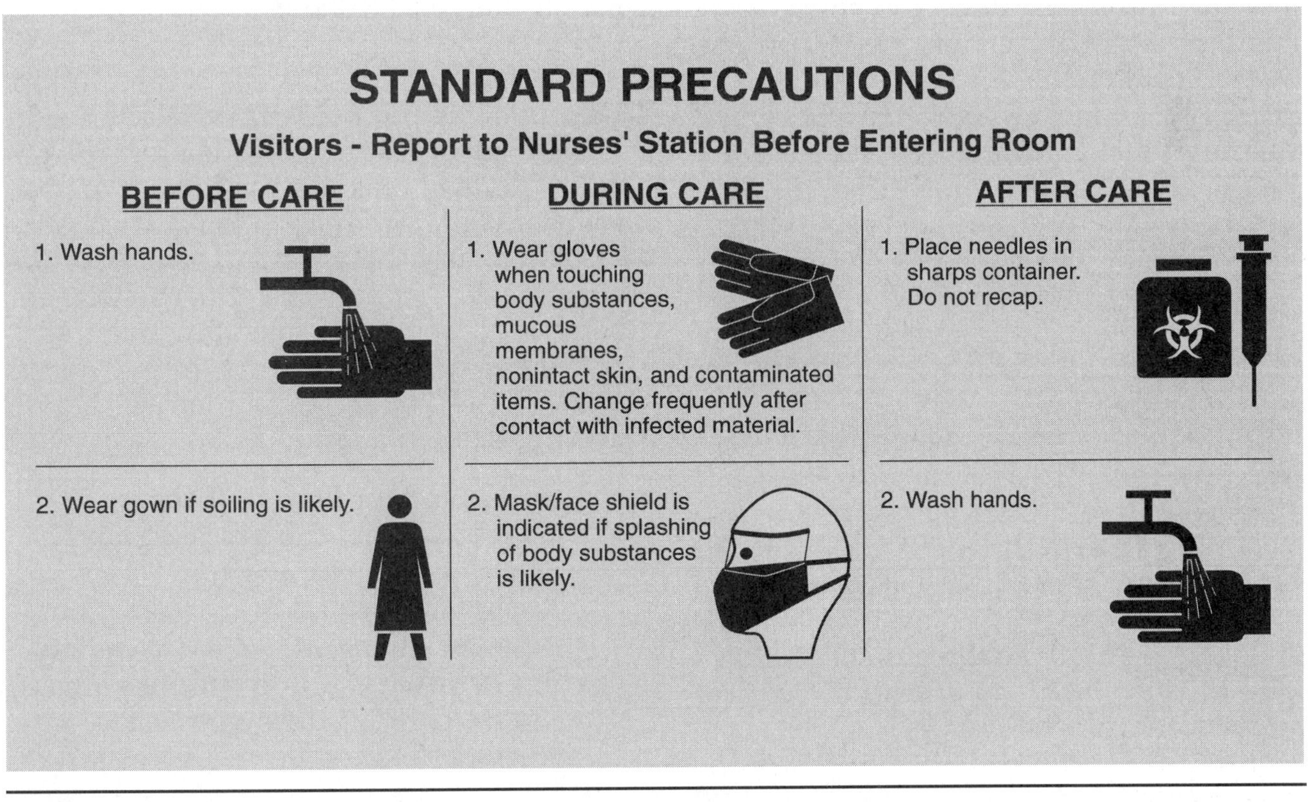

FIGURE 4-4
Standard precautions are used in the care of all residents regardless of disease or diagnosis. (Courtesy of Briggs Corporation, Des Moines, IA (800) 247-2343.

when performing certain tasks. PPE is apparel that protects the health care worker from contracting a disease from a resident. PPE also protects the resident from contracting a disease from a microbe passed from the worker's hands or uniform.

Guidelines for Selection and Use of Personal Protective Equipment

Standard precautions are used any time the health care worker anticipates contact with blood or any moist body fluid (except sweat), secretions, and excretions. They are also used any time you expect direct mucous membrane contact. Mucous membranes are found in the eyes, nose, mouth, and genital area. If either you or the resident has nonintact or broken skin, PPE must be used for contact. There are many variables in resident care situations, so there are no absolute guidelines available for the use of PPE. You must think about the situation and use good judgment. You are responsible for applying the principles of standard precautions and selecting the PPE according to the task. Equipment is worn during some direct resident care activities. For the most part, PPE is not necessary for feeding stable residents in the dining room. However, PPE must be worn during cleaning procedures when contact with blood, body fluids, secretions, or excretions is likely.

PPE will only protect you if it fits properly, it is free from defects, and you use it regularly and correctly. Never use equipment that is torn or has defects. Study and learn the principles of standard precautions so you can apply them correctly. This will protect you and facility residents. Always follow your facility's infection control policies and procedures.

Exceptions to the rules. Some facilities are teaching personnel from nonnursing departments to assist with feeding residents. This may result in exceptions to the usual infection control and barrier precautions rules. Traditionally, health care personnel keep clean and dirty (soiled or contaminated) persons and equipment separated. Because of this, nursing (and other) personnel cannot enter the kitchen. This reduces the risk of accidentally introducing potentially harmful germs into the food supply. There is usually no crossover between the laundry and housekeeping departments into nursing activities for the same reason. The objective is to keep from introducing harmful germs into resident care areas. Remember, germs can be on your clothing and in your hair, in addition to being on your hands.

There may be times when personnel from housekeeping and laundry departments are asked to assist with feeding residents. This makes sense in facilities that stop all cleaning when meal trays are on the units. (This is done to prevent the spread of germs.) It may be essential during staffing emergencies, such as a snowstorm. Your facility infection control committee may address this issue. If so, follow their policies and guidelines. In any event, it is probably not a good idea for personnel who have cleaned isolation rooms or washed isolation linen to assist with feeding. Schedule these activities to be done after meals, if necessary. Suggestions for personnel from housekeeping, laundry, and other areas who work in less clean parts of the facility to implement before feeding residents are:

- Pull long hair back and secure it with a hair tie or barrette or cover it with a disposable cap.
- Remove rings and other jewelry. Pin them to your uniform with a safety pin or place them in a secure area. Leave them off until you have finished feeding the residents.
- If you are wearing long-sleeved clothing, push the sleeves up or roll them up to the elbow. Leave them

up until you have finished feeding the resident.

- Wash your hands and forearms up to the elbows. Pay special attention to the areas between the fingers and the nail beds. Use a nail brush, if available. This is a more thorough handwashing than normal. It should take a minute or more. Take your time and make sure you wash all exposed surfaces of the hands and forearms.
- Cover your uniform with a clean resident gown, cloth or plastic apron, or smock. An isolation gown is not necessary unless needed to cover long-sleeved clothing. A cloth isolation gown works well for this purpose. You may also use a clean, long-sleeved lab jacket or coat. Button the lab coat to cover your uniform. If used, a lab coat should be worn only when feeding the resident, then removed.
- When you have finished feeding the resident, remove the gown and place it in the laundry. Gowns should be washed after each meal. Wash your hands again before returning to other duties.

Rules for Standard Precautions

Certain common procedures apply to using standard precautions in resident care. You must anticipate and select the correct type of personal protective equipment and wash your hands before and after every procedure.

Handwashing. Handwashing is done before all resident care and procedures. It is also done before applying and after removing gloves. Although gloves are worn, picking up a microbe on your hands is possible. This is because gloves may have microscopic defects. It is also possible to contact microbes unknowingly when removing gloves.

Barrier precautions. Personal protective equipment is also called barrier equipment. Using barrier precautions involves wearing gloves for handling or touching blood, any moist body fluid (except sweat), secretions, excretions, mucous membranes, and nonintact skin. If your gloves become visibly soiled or torn, you should remove them, wash your hands, and apply a clean pair of gloves. Change gloves:

- before each resident contact
- after each resident contact
- *immediately* before touching mucous membranes
- *immediately* before touching nonintact skin
- after you touch blood, body fluids, secretions or excretions, mucous membranes, or nonintact skin; before moving to care for another part of the body; or before touching clean equipment, supplies, or the environment
- after touching contaminated environmental surfaces or equipment
- any time your gloves become visibly soiled or torn

Your facility is required to have barrier equipment available in a variety of sizes in locations where use can be reasonably anticipated. Use gloves when necessary, but do not use them for all resident contact. *Using gloves at all times sends a negative message. It says that the resident is untouchable. Touching is important to all human beings, and residents need this contact.*

A gown (Figure 4-5) is worn any time your clothing may contact blood or any body fluids. The gown may be cloth or paper, but must be fluid-resistant. Many gowns are specially treated so they will

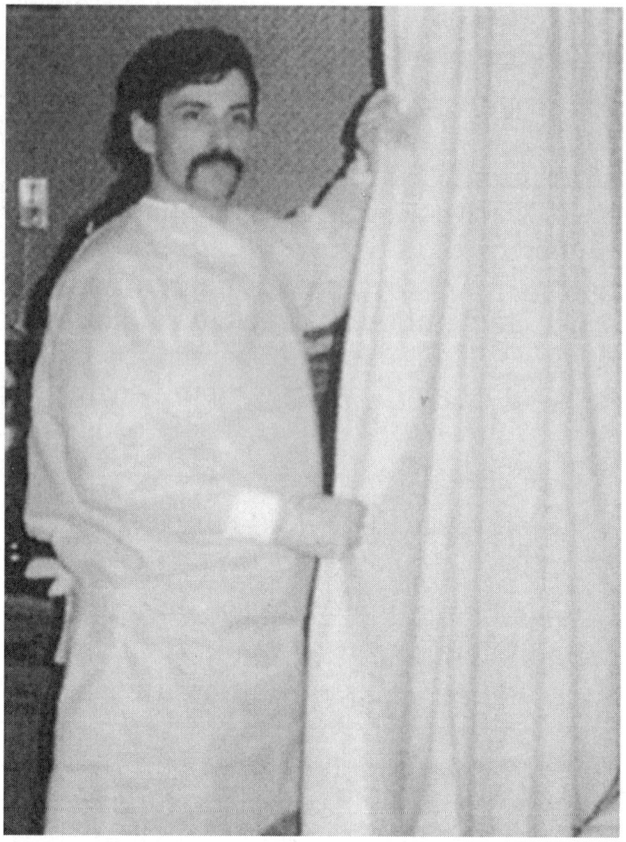

FIGURE 4-5
Wear a fluid-resistant gown if your uniform may have contact with blood, body fluids, mucous membranes, nonintact skin, secretions, or excretions.

resist fluid. The gown should cover your clothing and exposed areas of your body completely.

A face shield or goggles and a mask are worn during procedures when body fluids or secretions might splash on your face. A good rule to follow is that you can wear a mask without eye protection, but you should never wear eye protection without a mask. The facial barriers protect the mucous membranes in your eyes, nose, and mouth. You must anticipate what you will need and apply it before you begin a procedure. Check the equipment before using it. If it is cut or torn, it will not protect you and should be replaced. If you tear your gloves during a procedure, remove them as soon as possible. Wash your hands and put on a new pair of gloves before continuing.

PPE is discarded, laundered, or decontaminated according to facility policy after use. Be sure to replace what you have used so it is available the next time it is needed.

Procedure 2—Applying and Removing Gloves

Applying Disposable Gloves

1. Wash your hands.
2. Remove clean gloves from the box.
3. Put hands into the gloves, adjusting the fingers for comfort and fit.
4. Pull the cuffs of gloves up and adjust them over your wrists.

Removing Disposable Gloves

1. Grasp the outside of the glove on the nondominant hand at the cuff. Pull the glove off so that the inside of the glove faces outward (Figure 4-6A). Avoid touching the skin of your wrist with the fingers of the glove.
2. Place this glove into the palm of the hand that is still gloved.
3. Put the fingers of the ungloved hand *inside* the cuff of the gloved hand. Pull the glove off (Figure 4-6B) inside out. The first glove removed should be inside the second glove (Figure 4-6C).
4. Discard gloves in a covered container, according to facility policy.
5. Wash your hands.

Handling sharps. Handle sharp objects with care. If you must clean up broken glass, always wear gloves. Avoid picking up glass with your hands. Use a broom and dustpan (Figure 4-7A), forceps, or other mechanical method. Protect your hands from being cut. Dispose of broken glass and other sharp objects in a

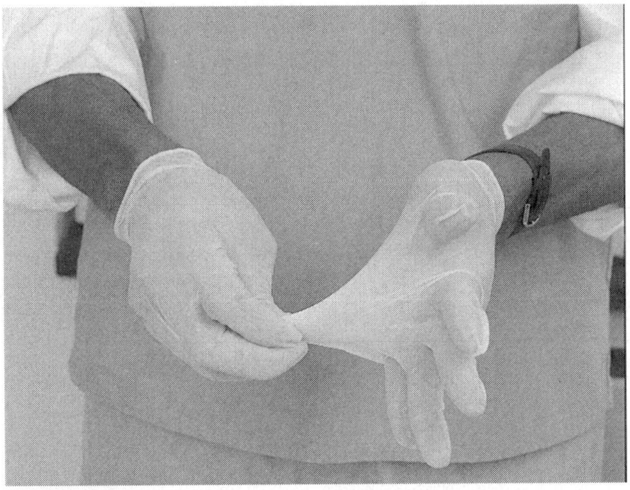

FIGURE 4-6A
Grasp the outside cuff of the glove without touching your hand.

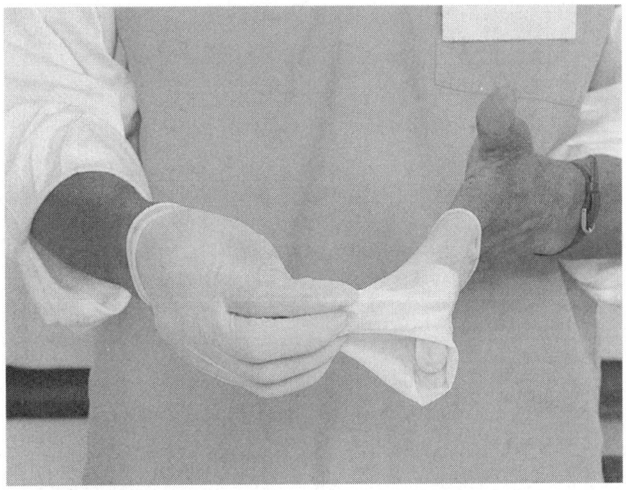

FIGURE 4-6B
Pull the glove off inside out. Hold it in the gloved hand.

puncture-resistant sharps container (Figure 4-7B).

Cleaning up blood and body fluid spills. Follow your facility's policy for cleaning up body fluid, such as urine on the dining room floor. In general, you should avoid mopping when residents are eating, as swinging a mop back and forth may move germs about. Many facilities apply absorbent powder to soak up the fluid, then cover the spill well with paper towels. (Place a wet floor sign.) After the fluid has been absorbed, sweep it up (Figure 4-8). Wipe the area with a facility-approved disinfectant.

Cleaning equipment. Each facility has policies and procedures for cleaning equipment. Utility gloves are better for cleaning duties than the disposable gloves used in resident care. The chemicals used for cleaning enlarge the pores of the disposable gloves. Although you probably cannot see this defect, the large pores will allow microbes to pass through.

Latex allergies. Some health care workers develop allergies to latex because of repeated exposure to latex gloves and other supplies. The powder in the gloves absorbs latex proteins. When the gloves are removed, the particles are inhaled, increasing sensitivity. Avoiding powdered gloves can decrease the risk of latex sensitivity. If you are allergic to latex, your facility will provide you with another type of glove. Glove liners and topical barrier

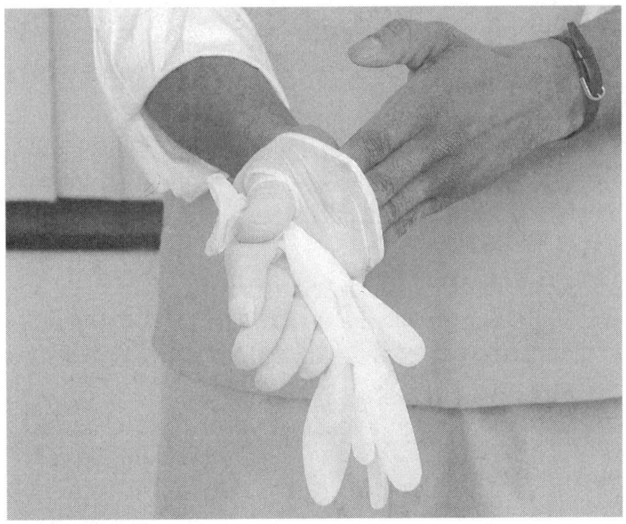

FIGURE 4-6C
Remove the opposite glove inside out. Discard your used gloves in a covered container, or according to facility policy.

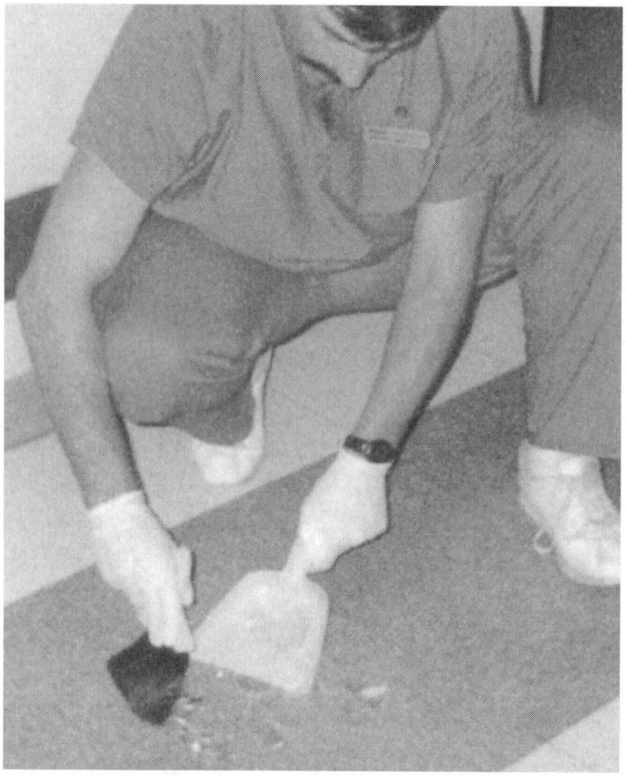

FIGURE 4-7A
Never pick up broken glass with your bare hands. Always wear gloves and use an instrument to clean broken glass, even if it is small.

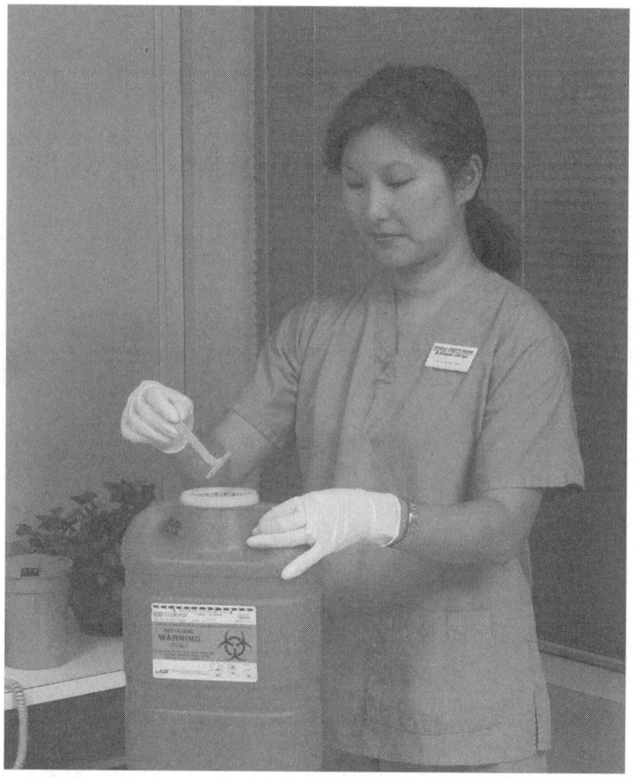

FIGURE 4-7B
Discard broken glass and all other potentially hazardous sharp objects in the puncture-resistant sharps container.

products are also available to individuals allergic to latex. The liner or topical product forms a barrier and prevents the latex from touching the skin.

CHAPTER REVIEW

Multiple Choice

Select the one best answer.

1. Normal flora:
   a. are harmful in areas where they do not belong.
   b. are practices used to prevent the spread of infection.
   c. are never harmful.
   d. are part of the chain of infection.

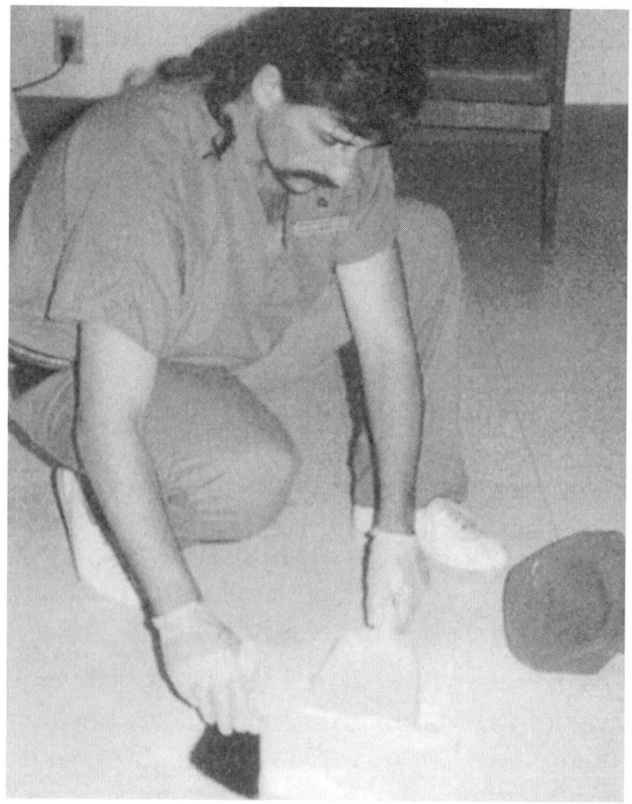

FIGURE 4-8
The absorbent powder turns the body fluid spill into a solid material for easy clean-up. The floor must be disinfected after the powder is removed.

2. Infections can be spread by all of the following *except:*
   a. direct contact.
   b. inhaling a microbe.
   c. touching a surface.
   d. vaccinations.
3. An example of common vehicle method of transmission is:
   a. touching a contaminated object.
   b. eating contaminated food.
   c. inhaling droplets in the air.
   d. mucous membrane contact with blood.
4. Droplets usually are confined to a space within:
   a. 3 feet of the resident.
   b. 6 feet of the resident.
   c. the facility ventilation system.
   d. the infected resident's unit.
5. The six factors necessary for an infection to spread are called the:
   a. mode of transmission.
   b. reservoir of infection.
   c. portal of exit.
   d. chain of infection.
6. _________ _________ must be used in the care of all residents.
   a. Standard precautions
   b. Susceptible techniques
   c. Normal flora
   d. Utility gloves
7. The most important measure health care workers use to prevent the spread of infection is:
   a. wearing a mask.
   b. disinfection.
   c. handwashing.
   d. wearing a gown.
8. Handwashing should be done:
   a. when coming on duty and when leaving at the end of the day.
   b. before picking up used (soiled) food trays.
   c. after applying and removing gloves.
   d. before clearing the dining room tables.
9. Handwashing should be done for a minimum of:
   a. 3 seconds.
   b. 5 seconds.
   c. 10 seconds.
   d. 15 seconds.
10. The most important part of the handwashing procedure is:
    a. using plenty of soap.
    b. using very hot water.
    c. using friction.
    d. keeping the fingers pointed down.
11. Gloves should be worn when:
    a. feeding each resident.
    b. picking up used meal trays.
    c. serving food trays.
    d. you have chapped hands.

UNIT 5

Safety and Emergencies

OBJECTIVES

- Spell and define key terms.
- Describe measures to take to keep the environment safe.
- List the three elements necessary for a fire to start.
- Describe what to do if you find a resident in an emergency situation.
- List seven guidelines to follow in an emergency.
- List the rules for using good body mechanics.
- Demonstrate care of the resident with choking and aspiration.
- Demonstrate care of the resident with an airway obstruction.

THE IMPORTANCE OF SAFETY IN THE LONG-TERM CARE FACILITY

Physical and mental changes occur with aging and in certain diseases. Many of these changes affect the residents' safety, awareness of hazards, and judgment, increasing the risk of incidents. Take safety seriously. This will keep your facility in compliance with the various agencies that inspect it, as well as protect employees and residents from injury.

Safety is everyone's concern. Every employee is responsible for keeping the environment safe and preventing **accidents**. Accidents are unexpected events that often result in injuries, which can range from minor to serious. An **incident** is an occurrence that disrupts the normal procedures and routine of the facility. A fall is an accident, but it is also an incident. If a resident wanders away and returns unharmed, an incident has occurred. This is not an accident. The nurse completes an incident report on all accidents and incidents. The report states exactly what happened, describes injuries, lists witnesses, and includes special notifications. Information written on the incident report is always **factual**. This is information that you *know* is true, not what you *think* may have happened. The resident is monitored for at least 24 hours or until problems related to the incident are **resolved**. This means the nurse believes the resident is stable and out of danger.

Providing a Safe Environment

The most common accidents in long-term care facilities are falls and burns. Most accidents can be prevented. Everyone benefits from a safe environment. You can do many things to make the facility safe. If you notice an unsafe condition that you can correct, do so immediately. Report unsafe conditions that you cannot correct to the nurse or proper person. Remind residents about safety. For example, a resident does not chew well and usually swallows large pieces of meat, such as half a hot dog. Remind and prompt him or her to chew well. Cut the meat into small pieces if you are feeding the resident. Follow the care plan for other approaches, such as alternating liquids with solids. If you discover a problem, such as loose **dentures** (false teeth), or the resident complains of painful teeth, promptly inform the nurse. Other things you can do to provide a safe environment are:

- Warn others of safety hazards.
- Follow safety policies and procedures.
- Set a good example by using safe practices.
- Attend classes on safety and practice what you learned.
- Monitor residents for safety problems; correct them or inform the nurse.
- Wipe up spills promptly, and place a "wet floor" sign (Figure 5-1). Pick up items left on the floor.
- Make sure there is a pathway for residents to walk through. Residents are more likely to fall if there is an obstacle course.
- Never run in the hallways.
- Remind residents to use the handrails.

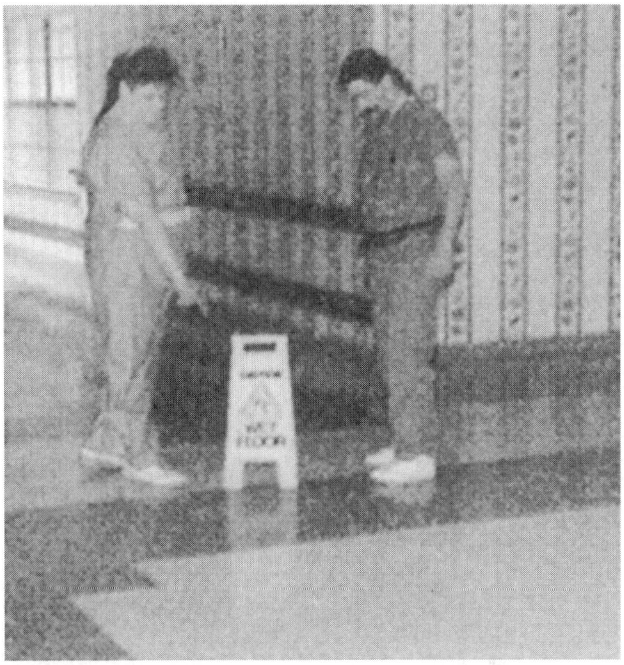

FIGURE 5-1
Promptly place a wet floor sign to warn others of slippery spots.

- Watch where you are going when pushing equipment or wheelchairs. Stop and look before going around corners or through doors. Take care when approaching or going through swinging doors.
- Avoid blocking exit doors or automatic fire doors with pieces of equipment or furnishings.

Safe use of chemicals. Many different types of **chemicals** are used in health care facilities. Chemicals may be harmful if they touch the skin or mucous membranes, or if they are swallowed or inhaled. Most cleaning products are chemicals. For chemical safety:

- All chemicals must have a clear label. Do not use the product if the label is not legible.
- Never pour chemicals into an unmarked container. Never use the contents of an unmarked container.

- Use chemicals according to the directions on the package.
- Keep cleaning products and other chemicals in a locked area when not in use.
- Never store chemicals in the same area as food or beverages.
- If you are using a cleaning product in a resident care area, you must be able to see it at all times. *Never put a bottle down and turn your back.*

The long-term care facility is required to keep **material safety data sheets (MSDS)** for all chemicals used. Your facility will teach you how to use the MSDS. Know the location of the MSDS. They will provide information and instructions for safe use, identify health risks, and describe first aid and safety precautions.

Safety and mentally confused residents. Besides the safety practices already discussed, keep sharp objects, small items that could be swallowed, and plants away from residents who are mentally confused. Check with the nurse if you are not sure about the safety of an item.

Equipment safety. You will push carts, operate appliances, and use the ice machine. Facilities have many electrical and mechanical devices. You should:

- Use your body correctly when bending, lifting, or moving equipment.
- Use equipment only according to manufacturers' directions.
- Follow facility policies and procedures for safe use of an item.
- Use electrical or mechanical equipment only as intended. For example, do not heat wet washcloths in the microwave to wipe residents' faces and hands after meals. Use warm water instead. (Get warm water from a resident care area. Do not use warm water from the kitchen.)
- Do not use electrical or mechanical equipment unless you have been taught how to use it safely.
- If you feel that an electrical item is unsafe, notify the proper person. Many facilities use a **lockout-tagout** system. A locking device is placed on the item in a way that prevents it from being used.
- Follow facility policies for reporting and removing unsafe or broken items from service.

Resident Identification Systems

Health care facilities use identification systems to alert employees to resident identities, special needs, and **risk factors**. Risk factors are conditions that suggest a problem *may* develop. Identifying risk factors and planning preventive care are key nursing functions. The presence of a risk factor does not mean a complication will develop. Once the risk is known, nursing personnel plan care designed to reduce or minimize the risk, thus preventing the complication. Most facilities use a system of colors, symbols, emblems, or designs that have special meaning to alert personnel to certain risk factors. The meaning and purpose of the system are known only to the employees. The risks are confidential, so the key to the systems used is not known to the residents, visitors, or public.

Many facilities use an **identification band** system. A plastic band is placed around the wrist or ankle listing identifying information, such as the resident's name, room number, and physician. Some facilities use color-coded identification bands for specific purposes. For example, a facility may use pink or red bands to identify residents with diabetes. Residents at risk of wandering outside may have a special color band. Some facilities do not use identification bands on residents. Residents are identified by sight only. The facility usually has a photograph of each resident. You must learn your facility policies for special alerts and for identifying residents. Always identify residents before feeding them or giving care. Check the resident's identification band (if present), and call the resident by name. Some residents will answer to any name they are called, so make sure that you have the correct resident. Do not be embarrassed if you have to ask a resident his or her name. It is better to ask than to provide care to the wrong resident.

Some facilities use self-adhesive colored dots on the bands. Dots may also be placed on the resident's diet card. The dots have special meanings. For example, a blue dot may identify residents who need extra liquids, or a red dot for a high-risk condition, such as choking. Find out the meaning of these systems, if used by your facility.

Some facilities use special wristbands for residents who may be in danger if they wander away. The bracelets contain magnetic sensors similar to those used in stores to prevent shoplifting. The resident may move freely about the facility. If he or she approaches an outside door or unsafe area, an alarm will sound. Facilities may also place an identifying object on a wheelchair, door frame, or elsewhere indicating the resident is at risk of falls. All staff are responsible for visually monitoring residents who wander and are at risk for falls.

Many facilities place the resident's name on the room door. Special decorations, such as bows or decorated hats, may also be used. These things help confused residents find their rooms. They are directed to find the "blue bow" or the "yellow hat."

Sometimes facilities have special emblems, such as pictures of leaves falling off a tree to indicate residents are at risk of falling. These pictures may be placed over the bedroom door or near the dining table. Facilities also use special color codes in the dining room, such as colored napkins. The color of the napkin will identify residents with special diets, nutritional problems, or needs.

Burn Prevention

Burns are a leading cause of injury. Residents with some diseases do not feel heat as acutely. Occasionally, a resident spills hot liquids, resulting in burns. Unsafe cigarette smoking is also a leading cause of burns. Know and follow your facility's policy for cigarette smoking. If you smoke, do so only in designated areas. Some facilities allow smoking outside. Others do not allow smoking anywhere on the property. Most facilities do not allow residents to keep smoking materials. They require staff to issue and light cigarettes and supervise residents when they smoke. Residents are not allowed to smoke in their rooms except in special circumstances, and then only with direct supervision. In any event, residents must smoke only in a supervised, designated smoking area or outside. Provide large, deep ashtrays for residents to use. Empty ashtrays only in metal cans with lids.

Thermal burns. **Thermal burns** are common injuries in long-term care facilities. Thermal burns are caused by contact with a hot substance, object, or open flame. Be sure that you do not serve very hot food or liquids to residents. If in doubt, place a drop of the food or liquid on your wrist to check the temperature. Help residents who are confused or who have poor hand control. Do not place hot items in front of them and walk away. Thermal burns are also caused by water that is too hot and careless smoking.

FIRE SAFETY

Long-term care facilities are built with safety features that will prevent fires from spreading. These include doors that close automatically when the fire alarm sounds, an automatic sprinkler system, smoke

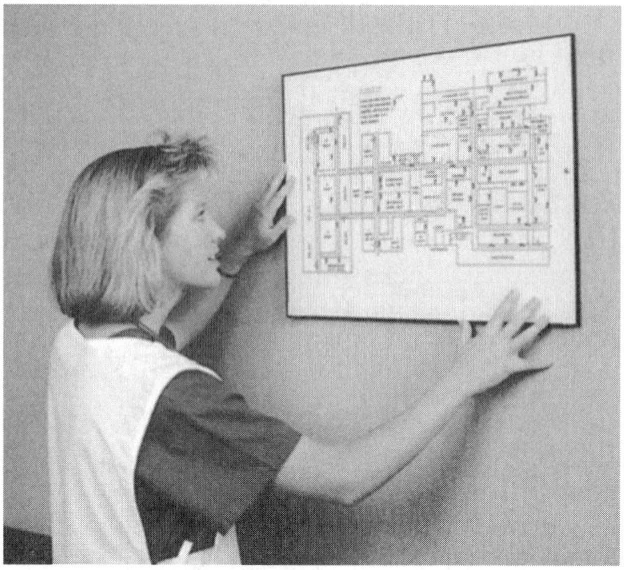

FIGURE 5-2
Become familiar with the facility evacuation plan and locations of exits.

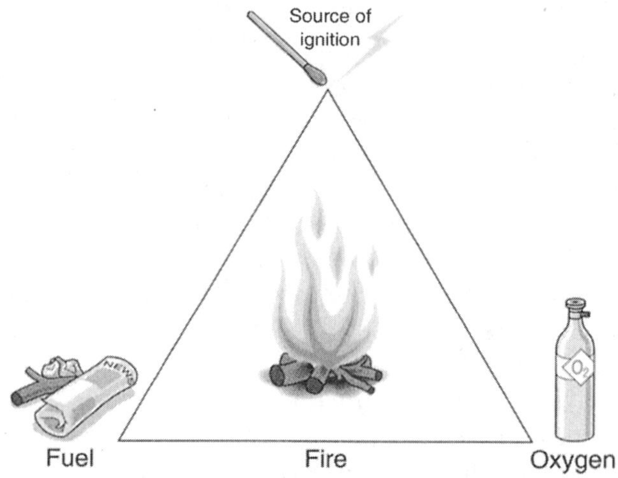

FIGURE 5-3
Three elements necessary to start a fire. Two of three are always available. You must prevent the source of ignition from contacting the others.

detectors, and fire exits. The materials used for the floors, doors, walls, and furnishings are fire-rated. This means they will take longer to burn. Despite the built-in safety features, facilities catch on fire. Fire alarms and extinguishers are located on the walls in the hallways. The facility will have an evacuation plan (Figure 5-2). Become familiar with the locations of alarms, extinguishers, and escape routes. Fire prevention is an important responsibility. Your facility will have periodic fire drills. Take them seriously. Your actions in a fire drill must become automatic, so you will react properly in a real fire.

The Fire Triangle

Three elements are necessary for a fire to start. These are oxygen, fuel, and a spark or source of ignition (Figure 5-3). Oxygen is in the air. Wood, paper, linens, and other materials provide fuel. Since two of the three elements necessary for fires are everywhere, the only thing missing is the spark, or source of ignition.

Steps to Take in a Fire Emergency

In a fire emergency remain calm and do not panic. Most facilities use the **RACE system** (Table 5-1). After the alarm has sounded, contain the fire by closing doors and windows. Move residents behind closed doors. Closing doors and windows slows the spread of fire. Clear hallways of residents and objects that will burn. If the fire is large and spreading rapidly, residents may be evacuated. Do not evacuate unless you are instructed to do so. If the fire is small, use a fire extinguisher to put it out. Fire extinguishers are used by aiming the spray at the base of the fire. The word PASS will help you remember how to use the fire extinguisher:

- **P** Pull the pin out of the upper extinguisher handle.
- **A** Aim the extinguisher at the base of the fire.
- **S** Squeeze the handle to discharge the contents of the extinguisher.

TABLE 5-1

STEPS TO FOLLOW IF YOU DISCOVER A FIRE	USING THE FIRE EXTINGUISHER
Follow the steps of **RACE**: **R** = ***Remove*** residents from the vicinity of the fire **A** = ***Activate*** the alarm **C** = ***Contain*** smoke and fire by closing doors and windows **E** = ***Extinguish*** the fire if it is small enough to contain and the proper equipment is available *or* **E** = ***Evacuate*** as directed by the fire department or person in charge	The **PASS** system is used to remember how to use the fire extinguisher: **P** = ***Pull*** the pin out of the handle **A** = ***Aim*** the extinguisher low, at the base of the fire **S** = ***Squeeze*** the extinguisher handle **S** = ***Sweep*** the extinguisher from side to side, aiming at the base of the fire

- **S** Sweep the extinguisher from side to side while keeping it aimed at the base of the fire.

In a fire, smoke is dangerous. Smoke rises, so more oxygen is available on the floor. If you can crawl to an exit, cover your mouth and stay on your knees. Before entering a room, touch the door with the *back* of your hand. *If the door is hot to touch, do not open it.* Opening the door could cause the fire to enter explosively. If the door is hot, stay there. Place wet blankets or towels under the door to keep smoke out.

OTHER EMERGENCIES

When a natural disaster occurs, many people can be injured in a short period of time. Know what natural disasters are possible in your area and find out what evacuation or safety measures are used by your facility. The facility will have a disaster plan that describes what actions to take. Learn facility codes for emergencies, such as "Doctor Red" for fire and "Code Black" for tornado. Learning and practicing emergency procedures in advance is important. Always remain calm in an emergency. When an emergency occurs, follow the nurse's directions. Sometimes you must act before the nurse arrives to keep residents from serious harm.

Guidelines to Follow in All Emergencies

- If you discover an ill or injured resident, remain with the resident and call for help.
- Do not move residents who have fallen unless they are in immediate danger.
- Stay calm and do not panic.
- Start emergency measures that you are trained and qualified to do while waiting for help to arrive.
- Once the nurse arrives, do as he or she directs.
- Know the location of emergency equipment and supplies.
- Avoid contact with blood, body fluid, secretions (except sweat), excretions, mucous membranes, and nonintact skin. Know where personal protective equipment is kept, and use it. Report accidental contact with blood or any body substances to the nurse.

Caring for a Resident with Vomiting and Aspiration

Food and air enter the body through a shared passage in the mouth (Figure 5-4). The passage branches into two divisions

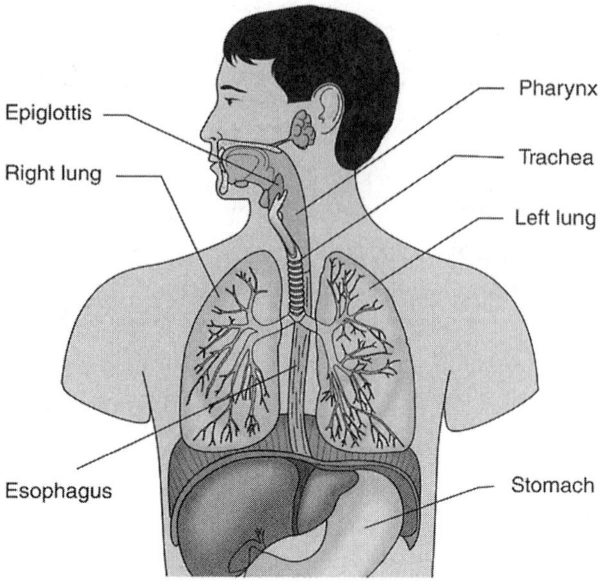

FIGURE 5-4
The trachea and esophagus share a common passage that food and air pass through in the throat. A muscular flap covers the trachea during swallowing to keep food from entering the lungs.

in the throat. Food goes into the esophagus, then to the stomach. Air goes into the trachea, then to the lungs. A small flap called the **epiglottis** covers the trachea when you swallow. This flap prevents food and liquid from entering the lungs. The ability to swallow is less efficient in persons with certain diseases and in persons who are elderly. Some residents pocket food in their cheeks. Food, water, or other objects may accidentally enter the trachea and lungs. This is called **aspiration**. It can occur when a resident is vomiting, bleeding, eating, or drinking. Thick secretions from the mouth may enter the lungs. Aspiration is serious. It can be prevented by turning the resident's head or body to the side if he or she vomits while lying down. Fluid cannot enter the lungs in this position.

Procedure 3—Emergency Care for Vomiting and Aspiration

1. Stay with the resident and call for help.
2. Apply gloves and other protective apparel, as needed.
3. Keep the resident's head elevated.
4. Keep the resident's body or head turned to the side to allow fluids to drain from the mouth.
5. Provide an emesis basin, plastic bag, or other container if the resident is vomiting.
6. Notify the nurse immediately if the resident:
   - is choking or unable to swallow
   - is unable to spit out the vomitus, blood, or secretions in the mouth
7. If the resident begins choking and an airway obstruction occurs, follow the procedure for clearing the obstructed airway.
8. Follow the nurse's instructions when he or she arrives.
9. Observe for and report to the nurse difficulty swallowing, bleeding, vomiting, choking, or aspiration.
   - Do not discard the vomitus until the nurse has seen it and obtained a specimen, if needed.
10. Dispose of items containing blood or other body secretions according to facility policy.
11. Remove gloves and dispose of them according to facility policy.
12. Wash your hands.

Dysphagia

Some residents have **dysphagia**, or difficulty swallowing food and liquids. This condition may occur in residents who have had a stroke or who have a condition of the nervous system. People who take medications that cause sedation or reduce saliva production are also at risk of dysphagia. You will not be asked to feed residents with known dysphagia. However, you may be feeding a resident in whom the problem is new or has not been diagnosed. Signs and symptoms of dysphagia are:

- taking a long time before beginning to swallow
- swallowing three or four times with each bite of food
- frequent throat clearing or coughing
- lack of a gag reflex or weak cough
- drooling or having difficulty controlling liquids and secretions in the mouth
- wet, gurgling voice
- refusing to eat, spitting food out, or pocketing food in cheeks
- unintentional weight loss
- tightness in the throat or chest
- feeling as if food is sticking in the esophagus or sternal area

If you observe any of these signs or symptoms, *stop feeding* the resident and inform the nurse. Residents with dysphagia are at high risk of choking and aspiration.

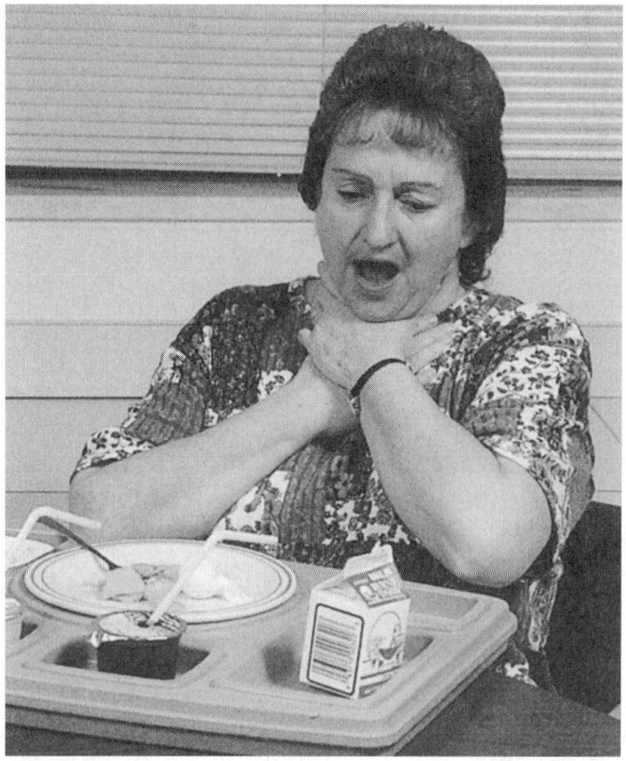

FIGURE 5-5
The universal choking sign. If a resident displays this sign, ask her if she can speak.

Caring for a Resident with an Obstructed Airway

Sometimes food or a foreign object is aspirated into the windpipe, or trachea. This causes an **obstructed airway**, which is a serious emergency. The resident will die if the obstruction is not removed immediately. When people are choking, they instinctively place one or both hands on the throat. This is known as the **universal choking sign** (Figure 5-5). If you see a resident with hands on the throat, ask if she can speak. If so, the airway is not obstructed. Stay with her and see if she can expel the object on her own. If the resident cannot speak, cough, or breathe, you must act immediately. The purpose of this procedure is to remove a foreign object from the airway of a conscious adult. The procedure is different for infants, small children, pregnant women, and unconscious adults.

Procedure 4—Emergency Care for Clearing the Obstructed Airway in a Conscious Adult Who is Sitting or Standing

Note: Never perform this procedure until you have been taught by a qualified instructor. It is recommended that you complete an approved course, taught by an American Heart Association or American Red Cross approved instructor. The information in this book is not intended to take the place of an approved course.

1. Ask the resident, "Are you choking?" or "Can you speak?"
2. If the resident can speak or cough, leave her alone and see if she can cough the obstruction out. Assist the resident if the cough is weak and ineffective and the resident is in obvious distress.

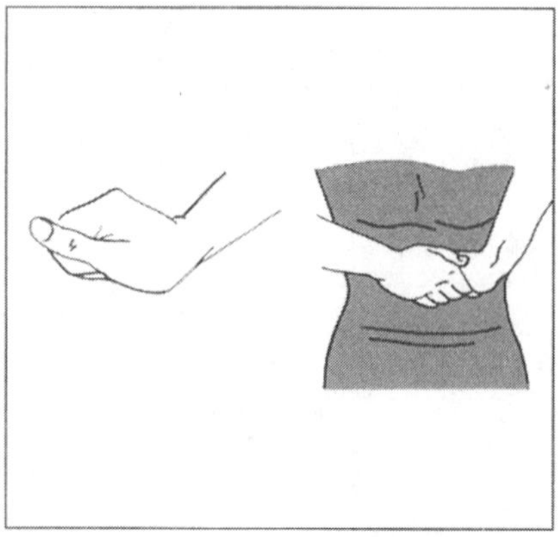

FIGURE 5-6A
Place your arms around the abdomen, slightly above the waist. Avoid resting your forearms on the ribs.

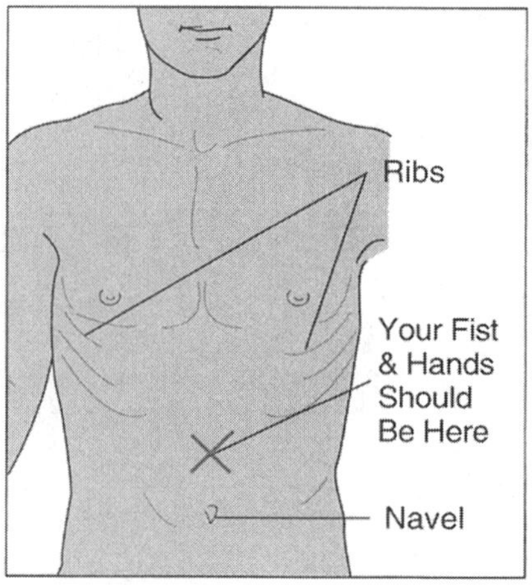

FIGURE 5-6B
Turn your thumb inward. Tuck it in so you can use your knuckle to compress the abdomen.

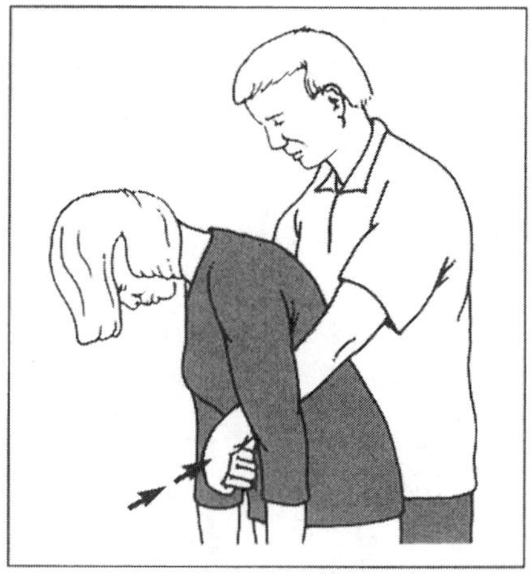

FIGURE 5-6C
Squeeze in and up. Each thrust is a separate and distinct movement designed to relieve the obstruction.

3. Stay with the resident and call for help.
4. Tell the resident that you will help.
5. Stand behind the resident and wrap your arms around her waist (Figure 5-6A).
6. Make a fist with one hand and place the thumb side of the fist against the abdomen, just above the navel (Figure 5-6B).
7. Grasp your fist with the other hand. Do not press on the ribs or breastbone with your forearms.
8. Squeeze inward and upward five times (Figure 5-6C). Each thrust should be a separate and distinct movement with the intent of removing the obstruction. You are trying to push the diaphragm up to force out the air behind the foreign body. As the air is expelled, it will push the object out.
9. If the resident does not expel the foreign body, repeat the inward, upward thrusts. If the resident begins to cough forcefully, wait and see if the object is expelled.
10. Repeat the abdominal thrusts until the object is expelled or the resident loses consciousness. Activate the emergency response system, if this has not already been done. Send someone else, if possible. Remain with the resident and continue to try to relieve the obstruction.
11. After the foreign body is expelled, stay with the resident and follow the nurse's directions.
12. Wash your hands.

PERSONAL HEALTH AND SAFETY

Stay home from work if you have a cold, flu, diarrhea, or other illness that may be infectious. Follow your facility's policy for reporting your absence. If you think you have been exposed to an illness at work, notify your supervisor and follow his or her instructions. To do your job well, you must be in good physical and emotional health. You will learn many health and safety principles and practices that you can apply to your personal life. Maintain your health by:

- practicing the principles of proper nutrition, good health, and personal hygiene.
- getting adequate rest; most people need eight hours of sleep each night.
- exercising for at least 30 minutes three times each week to stay healthy and relieve stress.
- seeing your doctor regularly for checkups and preventive health care. Treat medical problems early. Do not wait for them to become worse.
- practicing monthly self-examinations and having diagnostic tests recommended by your physician.
- getting immunizations, such as flu shots and others recommended by your physician to prevent disease.
- attending classes on health and safety.
- following facility policies and procedures for safety, and prevention of infection and injury.
- learning and following infection control techniques to prevent infection and disease.
- washing your hands (or using an alcohol-based hand cleanser) frequently throughout your workday and any time your hands are soiled.
- being nice to yourself, being aware of and meeting your own needs.
- using **good body mechanics** (Box 5-1) for bending, lifting, moving, and

BOX 5-1
Guidelines for Using Good Body Mechanics

- Keep your back straight.
- Your feet should be at least 12 inches apart.
- Avoid unnecessary bending at the waist and reaching.
- Face your work. Avoid twisting at the waist. Never lift and twist at the same time.
- Use smooth, even movements instead of quick, jerking motions.
- Before moving a heavy object, evaluate the load for weight and size. Ask for help, if needed.
- Before moving a heavy object, plan how you will do it.
- Take a deep breath before lifting. Exhale during the lift.
- Use the large muscles in your legs when lifting heavy objects.
- Bend from the hips and knees, never from the waist.
- Squat when lifting heavy objects from the floor.
- Tighten your abdominal muscles to support the spine.
- Avoid reaching for or lifting heavy objects that are above your shoulder height.
- Use both hands when lifting and moving heavy objects.
- Keep heavy objects as close to your body as possible when lifting, moving, and carrying.
- Push, pull, or slide heavy objects instead of lifting them whenever possible. Use your body weight to help you. Use a cart to push supplies instead of carrying them.
- Make sure you have a clear path. Before beginning, move or remove items and clutter on the floor.
- Turn your entire body instead of twisting your back or neck. If you must turn or change direction, take a few short steps or pivot instead.
- Ask for help from others if you are not sure whether you can move an object.
- Communicate well with others who are helping you. Synchronize your movement, such as "move on the count of three."

picking up items from the floor. Good body mechanics involves using your body correctly. Proper body mechanics means using the largest, strongest muscles to do the job. The strongest muscles are in your legs and arms. Your weakest muscles are in your back and abdomen. Practice good body mechanics until they become a habit. They will make your job easier, prevent fatigue, and reduce the risk of injury by making the best use of your strength and energy.

CHAPTER REVIEW

Multiple Choice

Select the one best answer.

1. Safety is the responsibility of:
   - **a.** the administrator.
   - **b.** the housekeeping department.
   - **c.** the maintenance department.
   - **d.** all employees.
2. Chemicals:
   - **a.** should be stored on the pantry shelf.
   - **b.** are not a concern in the long-term care facility.
   - **c.** may be repackaged into smaller containers, which are easier to handle.
   - **d.** should be locked in a cabinet or under visual control at all times.
3. The three elements necessary to start a fire are:
   - **a.** oxygen, fuel, and a spark.
   - **b.** oxygen, chemicals, and fuel.
   - **c.** matches, cigarettes, and chemicals.
   - **d.** lighter, matches, and nail polish remover.
4. If you find a resident who is ill or injured, you should:
   - **a.** Run and get the nurse.
   - **b.** Stay with the resident and call for help.
   - **c.** Call an ambulance immediately.
   - **d.** Ask another resident to get the administrator.
5. If you find a resident who has fallen on the floor, you should:
   - **a.** Help the resident back to bed.
   - **b.** Tell the resident she should have called for help before getting up.
   - **c.** Go to the desk and fill out an incident report.
   - **d.** Stay with the resident and provide emergency care that you are qualified to do.
6. The universal choking sign is:
   - **a.** one or both hands on the throat.
   - **b.** coughing and gagging.
   - **c.** turning blue in the face and neck.
   - **d.** waving your hands in the air.
7. An incident is a/an:
   - **a.** an unexpected event that results in injuries.
   - **b.** an occurrence that disrupts normal routines.
   - **c.** a fall or other serious injury to a resident.
   - **d.** an accident involving an employee.
8. Which of the following is true about incident reports?
   - **a.** Information written on an incident report must be factual.
   - **b.** Information written on an incident report must reflect your opinion.
   - **c.** The incident must be completely resolved before an incident report is done.
   - **d.** An incident report is completed only when a resident is injured.
9. The most common causes of injury in the long-term care facility are:
   - **a.** chemical ingestion and falls.
   - **b.** choking and electric shock.
   - **c.** burns and falls.
   - **d.** fires and natural disasters.
10. If you discover a fire, you should use the:
    - **a.** ABC plan.
    - **b.** PASS system.

c. PUSH system.
d. RACE system.

11. The codes for the facility identification systems are:
a. posted on the walls.
b. known only to employees.
c. used only by nurses.
d. a matter of public knowledge.

12. A risk factor:
a. indicates a problem will develop.
b. suggests a problem may develop.
c. is a concern only to nurses.
d. is a sign of serious illness.

UNIT 6

Good Nutrition

OBJECTIVES

- Spell and define key terms.
- Describe how nutrition influences health.
- List the categories in the food pyramid and give the number of daily servings from each.
- List five common categories of diets served in health care facilities.
- Describe problems that increase residents' risk for unplanned weight loss and malnutrition.
- Describe how to assist residents in meeting their nutritional needs.

THE IMPORTANCE OF GOOD NUTRITION

Nutrition is important to longevity and quality of life. Residents look forward to meals and snacks. For residents, eating is one of the most important activities of the day. Long-term care facility residents need good nutrition to maintain and restore their health, prevent disease and complications such as pressure ulcers, and promote healing. **Nutrients** are chemical substances in food that are necessary for life. The six nutrients that are essential for good health are listed in Box 6-1.

FOOD GUIDE PYRAMID

The U.S. Department of Agriculture (USDA) is a governmental agency that studies nutrition and makes recommendations. The USDA has grouped foods into six categories. They recommend that everyone eat a certain number of servings from each category every day. To refer to this information easily, the **food pyramid** (Figure 6-1) was developed to provide an easy-to-understand picture of daily nutritional requirements. The categories and USDA recommended servings are:

- bread, rice, cereal, and pasta group—6 to 11 servings a day
- fruit group—2 to 4 servings a day
- vegetable group—3 to 5 servings a day
- milk, yogurt, and cheese group—2 to 3 servings a day
- meat, poultry, fish, dry beans, eggs, and nuts group—2 to 3 servings a day
- fats, oils, and sweets—use sparingly

Eating according to the recommendations on the food pyramid will provide a well-balanced diet. Table 6-1 lists the portion sizes from each category. Because obesity

BOX 6-1

- **Vitamins**—organic compounds found in foods that perform vital functions and regulate processes in the body.
- **Minerals**—an essential part of all cells that contribute to the formation of the bones, teeth, and nails, and help rebuild body tissues.
- **Carbohydrates**—food products that provide fuel and energy for the body.
- **Proteins**—often called "nature's building blocks," proteins are essential for growth, healing, and good health.
- **Fats**—food products such as butter and oil, which are used as a source of energy and heat.
- **Water**—a liquid that is essential for life and health; water makes up 80% of body weight in infants. By late adulthood, approximately 40% of body weight is water. Water is very important for maintaining fluid balance, preserving essential minerals, and preventing major organ failure.

is a major public health problem, portion sizes are a serious concern. In 2004, the government announced its intention to revise the food pyramid because of growing problems with obesity in the United States. The new recommendations will not be known for several years.

Although the pyramid has six levels, the items in the small triangle at the top do not fit in any of the major food categories. The top of the pyramid is not considered a food group. The USDA recommends eating foods from the five major food groups shown in the three lower sections of the pyramid. Each of these food groups provides some, but not all, of the nutrients you need each day. Foods in one group cannot replace those in another. No single group is more important than another. For good health, you need them all.

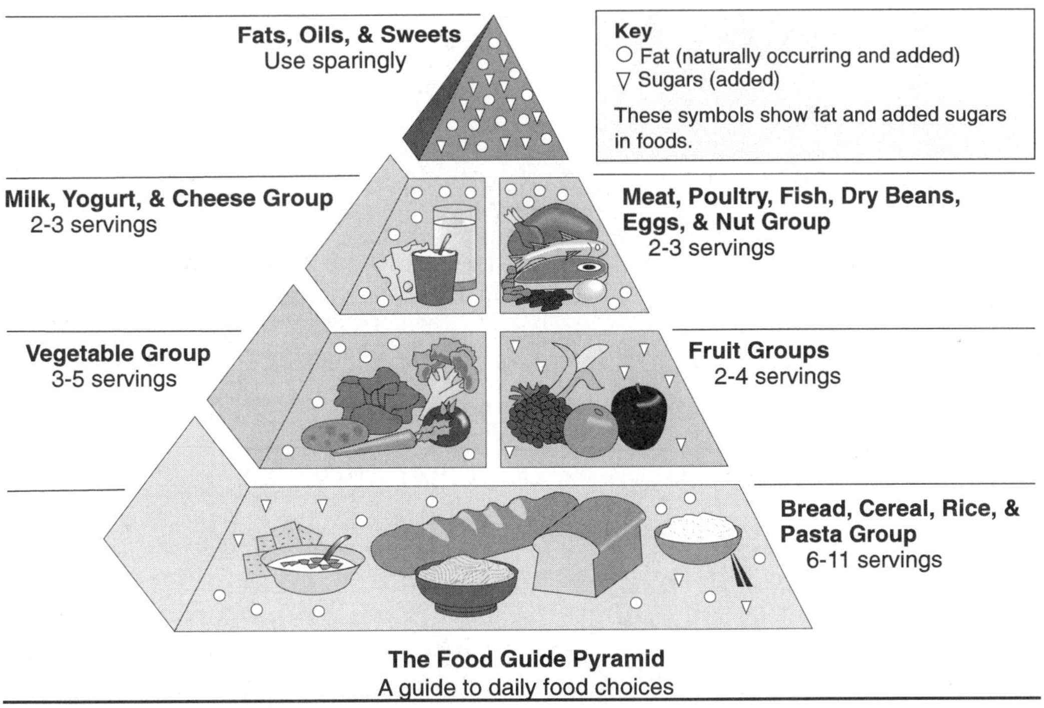

FIGURE 6-1
The USDA Food Guide Pyramid. (Courtesy of the U.S. Department of Agriculture).

TABLE 6-1

FOOD GROUP	ONE SERVING FROM THIS GROUP IS:
Bread, cereal, rice, and pasta group	1 slice of bread 1 tortilla ½ cup cooked rice, pasta, or cereal 1 ounce ready-to-eat cereal ½ hamburger bun, bagel, or English muffin 3–4 plain crackers 1 pancake (4 inch diameter) ½ large croissant ½ medium doughnut or danish 1/16 cake (average size cake) 2 medium cookies 1/12 of an 8″ pie
Vegetable group	½ cup chopped raw or cooked vegetables 1 cup raw, leafy vegetables ¾ cup vegetable juice ½ cup scalloped potatoes ½ cup potato salad 10 french fries
Fruit group	1 piece fruit or melon wedge ¾ cup fruit juice ½ cup chopped, cooked, or canned fruit ¼ cup dried fruit
Milk, yogurt, and cheese group	1 cup milk or yogurt 1½ ounces cheese (natural) 2 ounces cheese (processed) 1½ cups ice cream or ice milk 1 cup frozen yogurt
Meat, poultry, dry beans, eggs, and nuts group	2½ to 3 ounces cooked lean beef, pork, lamb, veal, poultry, or fish (a portion the size of a deck of cards)
	½ cup cooked beans, 1 egg, or 2 tablespoons peanut butter, or ⅓ cup of nuts equal 1 ounce of meat
Fats, oils, and sweets	Use sparingly

70+ Food Guide Pyramid

In 1999, researchers at the USDA's Human Nutrition Research Center on Aging at Tufts University, Boston, proposed changes to the food guide pyramid for adults age 70 and older (Figure 6-2). These changes make the food guide pyramid a more appropriate tool for elderly individuals, and are designed to help them optimize their food intake. Some dietitians use this food pyramid when planning meals for long-term care facility residents. Table 6-2 compares the two food pyramids. Facilities that use this pyramid usually provide water on resident food trays, or place a carafe on the tables in addition to the other beverages.

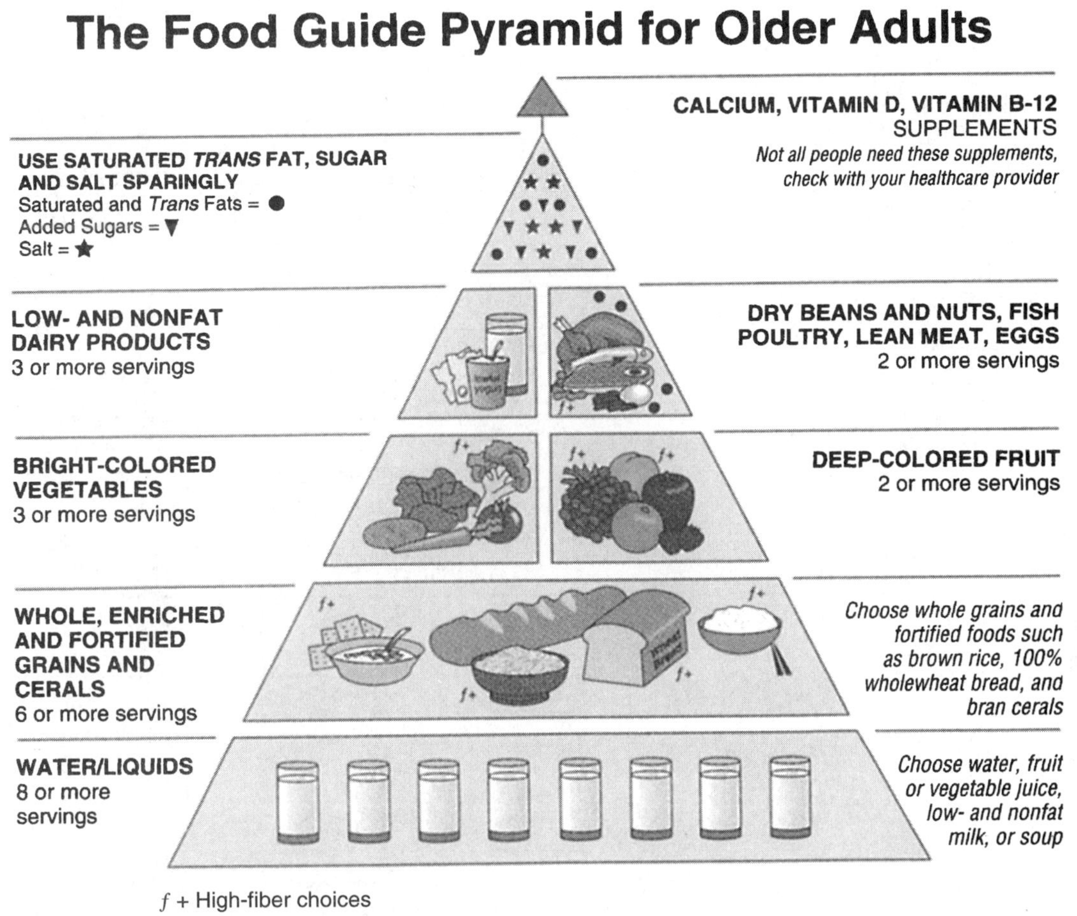

FIGURE 6-2
The Tufts University 70+ food pyramid. The liquid at the base of the pyramid is an important part of its structure. The liquids include water and any nonalcoholic, caffeine-free beverage. The fiber symbols throughout the pyramid remind the user to select foods that are high in fiber. (Courtesy of Tufts University).

MALNUTRITION AND UNPLANNED WEIGHT LOSS

Malnutrition is inadequate nutrition due to a poor diet or an inability to absorb nutrients. This is a serious condition that has dire complications. It can and does occur in long-term care facility residents, despite balanced diets and nutritional supplements. Mealtime is a busy time in the long-term care facility, especially on the day shift, when two meals are served. Some residents do not consume sufficient nutrients, although they are available. Some become frustrated and stop eating because feeding themselves is simply too difficult. Residents who are at greatest risk of malnutrition and unintentional weight loss are those who:

- cannot recognize or identify feelings of hunger or thirst
- need help eating and drinking
- eat less than half their meals and/or planned snacks
- are sad, have crying spells, or withdraw from others
- are confused, wander, pace, or have increased calorie needs because of activity

TABLE 6-2
USDA Food Guide Pyramid Compared with 70+ Food Guide Pyramid

USDA FOOD GUIDE PYRAMID	70+ FOOD GUIDE PYRAMID
	Adds a small supplement flag to the top, suggesting that supplements for three nutrients—vitamin D, calcium, and vitamin B12—may be appropriate for some, but not all individuals.
Fats, oils, and sugars used sparingly.	Fats, oils, and sugars used sparingly.
2 to 3 servings of milk	3 or more servings of milk. Low-fat products recommended.
2 to 3 servings of meat	2 or more servings of meat
3 to 5 servings of vegetables, 2 to 4 servings of fruits	3 or more servings vegetables, 2 or more servings of fruit. Fiber-rich, whole fruits and vegetables are recommended instead of juices. Deeply colored yellow, green, orange, and red fruits and vegetables are recommended, as well as vegetables like cabbage, cauliflower, and broccoli.
6 to 11 servings of grain-based food	Grain group 6 or more servings, emphasizing increased fiber and nutrient density.
	Eight 8 ounce glasses of water form the base of the pyramid. This includes any nonalcoholic, caffeine-free beverage. This is the most significant difference between the USDA pyramid and 70+ food guide pyramid. It emphasizes the importance of water for elderly adults.
	A fiber icon (f+) has been added for good sources of fiber. Fiber is important for elderly individuals.

- have diabetes, lung disease, cancer, HIV, or other chronic diseases
- forget what they ate, forget if they ate, or forget to eat altogether
- lose interest or become distracted before the meal is finished
- no longer know the purpose of food
- do not know what utensils are used for
- have mouth pain or unrelieved chronic pain
- have no dentures, or have dentures that do not fit correctly
- have difficulty chewing or swallowing or need to be prompted to chew and swallow
- have medical problems that make it difficult to get utensils or a cup to their mouth
- cough or choke while eating
- take certain medications
- have untreated (or ineffectively treated) depression

Barriers to good nutrition are both physical and mental. Medical problems and medications may also interfere with nutrient use. Residents on restricted diets and those who prefer ethnic and cultural foods may not eat enough. Young and middle-aged residents may prefer foods such as stir fry, sandwiches on pita bread, pizza, french fries, and tacos. These items are not routinely served in long-term care facilities. We have the freedom to eat what we want, when we want, where we want. Residents may not. The dietary department interviews residents concerning their food likes and dislikes. Honoring residents' food preferences is important. Inform the nurse if a resident expresses food likes or dislikes, or refuses to eat a certain item. Treating the resident's food choices as an inconvenience negatively affects the resident and adds to the feeling of living in an institution. Honoring food choices improves resident self-esteem and quality of life.

Unplanned weight loss can be a serious problem in ill and elderly persons. A resident who is losing weight is probably not receiving adequate nutrients. Lack of proper nutrients increases the risk of serious illness, infection, skin breakdown, and other conditions. Malnutrition is diagnosed based on weight loss and laboratory values. Laboratory values change when residents consume insufficient protein and calories. A lack of protein may cause the resident to develop **edema**, or swelling of the body. Abnormal blood pressure may develop. Because malnutrition is not diagnosed based on weight loss alone, obese and overweight residents may also become malnourished.

Other Factors Influencing Residents' Appetites and Ability to Eat

Food is much more than something to eat. Of course, we eat for pleasure and enjoyment. For most people, food is also love, security, and comfort. Positive and negative memories may be associated with food. Most family gatherings and activities involve food. Religious, ethnic, and cultural gatherings involve food. The appearance and smell of foods affect whether the resident accepts these items.

Many residents require assistance with meals because of physical and mental impairments. Some need prompting and coaxing. Ensuring that all residents receive adequate nutrition is a challenge. Food service is a great responsibility that is shared by many team members. Most residents with feeding problems have a special care plan to direct staff in promoting good meal intake. Follow the plan of care and the nurses' instructions. Observations, suggestions, and troubleshooting techniques that may assist in identifying and solving resident problems are listed below.

Staff must pay careful attention to:

- making food look and smell as attractive as possible
- serving meals promptly and maintaining proper food temperature
- creating a pleasant mealtime atmosphere
- providing adaptive devices and arranging the environment to promote feeding independence

Immobility, aging, and disease.

Many changes associated with the aging process, disease, immobility, and medications affect the resident's appetite. The most important of these are:

- Loss of appetite results from lack of activity, illness, pain, or boredom.
- Decreased saliva production causes difficulty with swallowing and digesting of starches, and increased risk for tooth decay.
- Taste buds on the tongue decrease, beginning with sweet and salt; changes in taste buds may result in appetite changes and increase in condiment use.
- Gag reflex is less effective, increasing the risk of choking.
- The ability to cough is less effective, resulting in pooling of secretions and fluid in the lungs, increasing the risk of infection and choking.
- Movement of food into the stomach through the esophagus is slower.
- Digestion of food in the stomach is slower, so food remains there longer before moving to the small intestine.

- Flatulence (gas) increases.
- Indigestion and slower absorption of fat result from decreased digestive enzymes.
- Food movement through the large intestine is slower, resulting in constipation.
- Delayed release of insulin increases blood sugar levels; the incidence of diabetes increases with age.
- Metabolism and body function slow, reducing the amount of calories needed for the body to function normally. This increases the risk of overweight and obesity.
- The sense of thirst is diminished with aging, and elderly individuals frequently do not take in sufficient fluids.

Environment. Appetite is affected by the environment. The OBRA 87 laws require facilities to maintain a homelike environment. This is particularly important in the dining room. A pleasant atmosphere improves residents' appetites. Tablecloths, centerpieces, attractive dishes, table decorations, and seasonal room decor promote good intake (Figure 6-3). Many residents enjoy quiet music and companionship at mealtime. Unpleasant odors and offensive behavior negatively affect the appetite. Managing problems immediately promotes a pleasant atmosphere. Knowing how the atmosphere affects residents is important. Quality of life is greatly affected by the quality of the mealtime experience.

Cognitive impairment. Residents with cognitive impairment are easily dis-

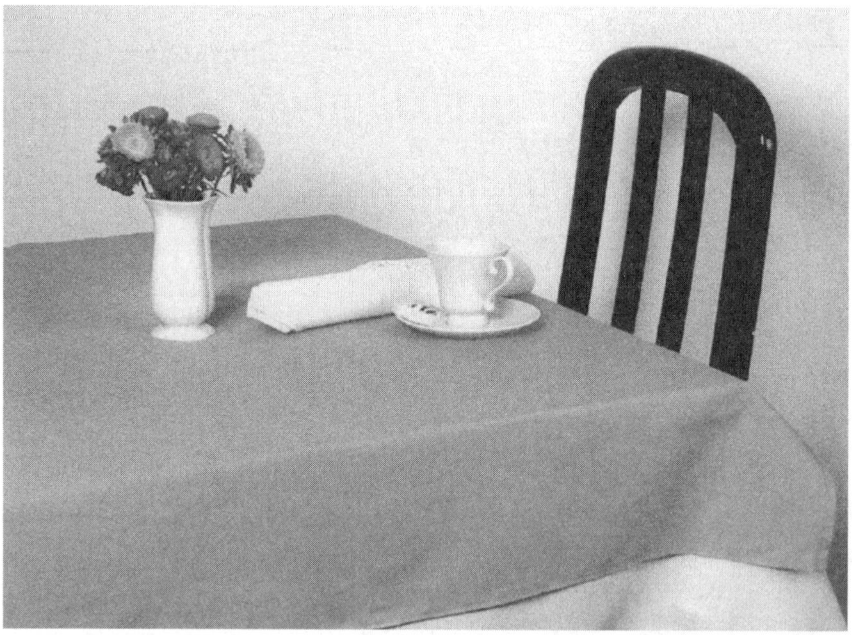

FIGURE 6-3
Serving meals involves more than putting food on plates. Creating an appealing atmosphere by using an attractive table setting, good lighting, flowers, tablecloths, and other steps can make meals more palatable. The atmosphere and environment in the dining room affect residents' appetites. Eating is a social occasion, and residents often eat better in groups in the community dining room setting. Staff should strive to make the dining experience pleasurable, preserve resident dignity, and accommodate preferences. A warm, comfortable, attractive dining environment that enables residents to maximize their potential usually enhances food and fluid intake. The results of one study suggest that residents with cognitive impairment eat better if food is served on bright-colored plates and glasses, such as deep blue or bright red. (Courtesy of Medline Industries, Inc. (800) MEDLINE.)

tracted and may not eat well. They are busy monitoring the activity in the room instead of eating. Some residents wander and cannot sit still through an entire meal. Approaches to assist this special group are discussed in the next unit.

HEALTH CARE FACILITY DIETS

Physicians write diet orders based on the residents' individual medical and nutritional needs. The dietary department prepares food served in the facility. A licensed dietitian writes the menus to be sure that diets are well balanced. The dietitian writes special menus for people with certain diseases to assure that the nutrients provided meet their needs. Enjoying food and drink is one of life's greatest pleasures. Facilities try to balance medical needs with quality of life needs. Diets are as liberal as possible, considering residents' conditions.

Many types of diets are served in long-term care facilities. Each facility has a listing of the types of diets served. Facilities post the menu each day. Some facilities have a menu, which enables residents to select what they want to eat. The common categories for diets served in long-term care facilities are:

- regular, or general diets
- liquid diets
- soft or bland diets
- mechanically altered diets
- therapeutic diets

Regular Diets

The **regular diet** is a normal, unrestricted diet. This diet is served to residents with no dietary restrictions. The diet is well balanced and has a variety of foods from the food pyramid.

Liquid Diets

Liquid diets are served to residents after surgery and before some tests. They are also used for residents who have nausea, vomiting, or diarrhea. They are not nutritionally complete and should only be used for a short time. The two main types of liquid diets are:

- **Clear liquid diet** (Figure 6-4). This diet is high in water and carbohydrates and consists of liquids that you can see through. It includes clear soda pop (seven up and ginger ale), broth, tea, soup, gelatin, popsicles, and strained fruit juices.

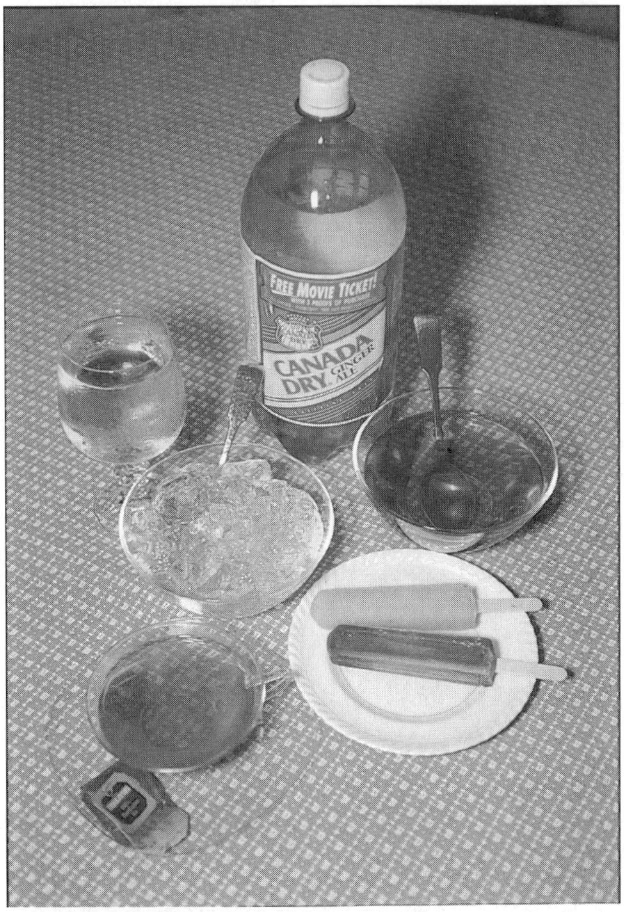

FIGURE 6-4
Items on a clear liquid diet include only liquids that you can see through.

- **Full liquid diet.** A diet consisting of all clear liquids plus milk-based liquids. It includes cream soups, milk, ice cream, eggnog, and yogurt.

Soft or Bland Diets

- **Soft** or **bland diets**. This diet is served to residents with digestive problems or those who cannot eat spiced or seasoned food. Seasoning is limited and the residue is low. Food includes soups, white meat and fish, cream cheese and cottage cheese, breads, crackers, and milk products.

Mechanically Altered Diets

Mechanically altered diets are served to residents who have chewing, swallowing, or digestive disorders. Any kind of diet can be blenderized to alter the mechanical consistency of the food. The two main types of mechanically altered diets are:

- **Pureed diet** (Figure 6-5). This diet is blended with liquid so the food is smooth without large particles. The food has the consistency of pudding or baby food, but should not be watery. If the diet is blended properly, a plastic spoon will stand upright in the food without falling over.
- **Mechanical soft diet**. This diet is usually served to residents with chewing problems. Meats and hard foods are ground to the consistency of hamburger. Soft items, such as bread, are not ground. The food is not reduced to liquid in this diet.

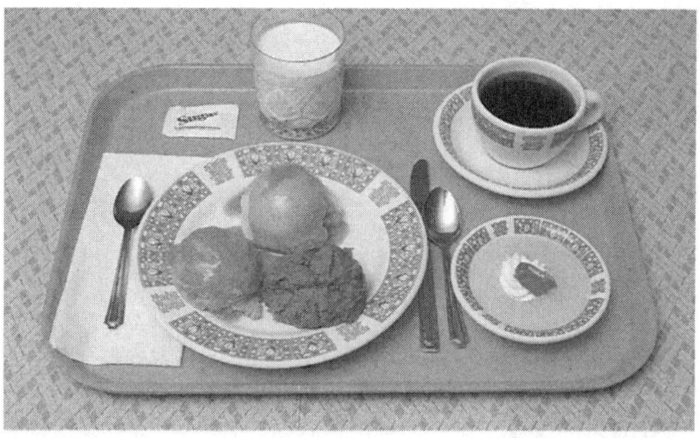

FIGURE 6-5
The pureed diet should have a firm consistency. Liquid should not run from the food.

Therapeutic Diets

Therapeutic diets are served to treat certain medical diseases or conditions. The dietitian plans these diets to meet residents' treatment needs. Regular food is used, but preparation may be different from a regular diet. For example, certain foods on a regular diet are prepared with salt. A resident on a salt-restricted diet would have the same food item prepared without salt. Each therapeutic diet has special requirements, and some foods may be restricted on certain diets. The common types of therapeutic diets are:

- **Diabetic diet**. A diabetic diet is served to residents with diabetes mellitus.
  - Some diabetic diets count calories.
  - The **no concentrated sweets** diet is commonly served to residents with diabetes. Concentrated sweets, such as sugar, canned fruits, and sweetened desserts, are restricted.
  - Normal foods are used, but food is prepared without free sugar.
  - Meals and snacks must be served regularly and promptly to maintain blood sugar. Some residents take medication to lower the blood sugar. If intake is inadequate, or meals are missed or delayed, the blood sugar may drop to critical levels. If a resident with diabetes does not eat, inform the nurse.

- **Calorie-controlled diet**. This diet is usually served to residents who are overweight.
  - This is a balanced diet, but portions of some foods are smaller than in regular diets.
  - Sugar and concentrated sweets are avoided.
- **Sodium-restricted diet**. This diet is served to residents with heart or kidney disease. The average American consumes 2 to 6 grams of sodium in food each day. Table salt is a major source of sodium in the diet.
  - The amount of sodium (salt) permitted each day is ordered by the doctor.
  - Salt substitutes may be used only with a physician's order.
  - Foods such as potato chips and snacks, ham, bacon, pickles, and some canned foods contain a large amount of sodium and should be avoided.
  - Sodium-restricted diets are some of the most difficult diets to follow.
- **Low-fat** and **low-cholesterol diet**. This diet is served to residents with heart, blood vessel, liver, and gallbladder disease.
  - Fats are limited or avoided
  - Baked or broiled lean meats, fruits, vegetables, and low-fat dairy products are served.

Other types of diets. Many other specialized diets can be served in long-term care facilities. Those listed here are most common and nonrestrictive. Residents have many unique needs, and other types of diets may be necessary. Some diets restrict fiber. Others increase or decrease protein. Some are high in calories. Some residents are on special diets because of religious prohibitions of certain foods.Special dietary requirements of cultural and religious groups are listed in Appendix A.

Large portions. Occasionally, a physician will write an order for "double portions" to increase a resident's food intake. This is a misnomer; "large portions" is probably more accurate. In most facilities, "double portions" is not a valid diet order, and the nurse usually contacts the physician and changes the order. To truly give double portions, the facility would have to double every food item on the tray, including milk, bread, and dessert. When a "large portions" order is written, two servings of the meat and vegetable are provided. Single portions of other food items are served. If you encounter a "double portions" order, clarify it with the nurse.

Lactose intolerance. **Lactose intolerance** is the inability to properly digest milk sugar, which is also called lactose. Signs and symptoms of lactose intolerance include abdominal bloating, cramping, gas, nausea, and diarrhea after eating dairy products. Pills are available to enable the resident to consume dairy products, and drops may be put in milk. Some individuals with lactose intolerance can eat yogurt and hard cheese without problems.

Food allergies. Allergies occur when you ingest a food, and your immune system reacts to it, believing it is a threat to your body. Your immune system tries to eliminate the invader by releasing chemicals that cause blood vessels to dilate and leak. Skin rashes, vomiting, and other side effects may occur. The reaction can be life-threatening. Nuts and milk proteins are common food allergies, but a resident may be allergic to any food substance. Take food allergies seriously. Avoid serving foods to which the resident is allergic.

Supplemental Feedings and Nourishments

Supplemental feedings and nourishments are served to meet special nutritional needs. Many residents have poor appetites, are underweight, or are at nutritional risk. Nourishments are given to maintain or increase weight. Common foods or beverages, such as milkshakes, ice cream, or juices, may be served. Some physicians order canned or packaged beverages, such as Ensure or Resource. A nutritional beverage is normally called a supplement. In most facilities, a physician's order is needed to provide supplements. If this is the case, the facility documents the percentage of supplement the resident consumes on a flow sheet. Supplements and nourishments should be served between meals. They are sweet, are filling, and will suppress the appetite if given with meals or immediately before meals.

Snacks. Most facilities offer snacks during the day or at bedtime. These are light food items, such as milk, juice, graham crackers, cookies, or fruit. Some facilities document snack intake, or whether the resident accepted or refused the snack item.

CHAPER REVIEW

Multiple Choice

Select the one best answer.

1. How many nutrients are essential for good health?
   a. two.
   b. three.
   c. five.
   d. six.
2. The type of food called "nature's building blocks" is:
   a. minerals.
   b. proteins.
   c. carbohydrates.
   d. vitamins.
3. According to the USDA food pyramid, how many servings of fruit should you have each day?
   a. 2 to 4.
   b. 3 to 5.
   c. 1 or 2.
   d. 6 to 11.
4. According to the USDA food pyramid, how many servings of bread, rice, cereal, or pasta should you have each day?
   a. 2 to 4.
   b. 3 to 5.
   c. 1 or 2.
   d. 6 to 11.
5. The 70+ food guide pyramid recommends:
   a. Eight 8 ounce glasses of water each day.
   b. Three to four servings of fiber daily.
   c. Two servings of vegetables daily.
   d. Restricting meat to 4 ounces daily.
6. Mr. Yore is on a full liquid diet. Which of the following would you expect to find on his tray?
   a. vegetable soup.
   b. pureed fish.
   c. yogurt.
   d. peach cobbler.
7. Therapeutic diets:
   a. are planned by the dietitian to meet special medical needs.
   b. are rarely served to elderly residents.
   c. have no effect on residents with heart disease or diabetes.
   d. are always limited in sugar and salt.
8. Foods that are high in sodium include:
   a. fresh fruit.
   b. fresh vegetables.
   c. bread and whole grains.
   d. lunch meat and ham.
9. The dining environment:
   a. does not affect quality of life.
   b. affects all residents.
   c. affects alert residents only.
   d. affects confused residents only.

10. Malnutrition:
- **a.** does not occur in the long-term care facility.
- **b.** is not a risk for overweight residents.
- **c.** may develop in elderly facility residents.
- **d.** is a problem only for residents who are confused.

UNIT 7

Assisting Residents with Meals

OBJECTIVES

- Spell and define key terms.
- Explain why satisfaction with meals is important to residents.
- Describe how to prepare the dining area and position residents for meals.
- List the guidelines for assisting residents in the dining room.
- Describe how to stimulate resident conversation.
- Demonstrate the technique for spoon-feeding a resident.
- Describe how to assist residents with problems that interfere with eating.
- Explain how to encourage and maintain resident independence with eating.
- State the purpose of adaptive devices.
- Define snacks, nourishments, and supplements and state when each is used.

IMPORTANCE OF FOOD

Quality of life in the long-term care facility is heavily dependent on the quality of food and meal service. Many residents look forward to meals. Although more study needs to be done on this area, we know that many resident complaints are received by surveyors concerning food service. Common complaints about food service are:

- clinical dining atmosphere that is not comfortable or homelike
- residents are unable to choose where they eat their meals
- residents are unable to make choices in their selection of food
- lack of good service
- lack of variety in the menu
- unappetizing appearance of food
- lack of seasoning
- failure to honor food preferences
- food temperatures not maintained
- not getting enough to eat

Making mealtime special is an important responsibility, and adding nutrition assistants is being done to enhance quality of life. Having friendly staff who show sincere concern for residents' welfare helps create a comfortable atmosphere at meals. If residents are satisfied with the quality of food and food service, they tend to view everything else in a positive light. Complaints do not necessarily reflect poor-quality food. They often reflect quality of life problems.

PREPARING FOR MEALS

Normal aging changes, illness, and certain medications can affect the resident's appetite. Make the environment and food as pleasant as possible. Prepare the dining area and residents in advance so meals can be served quickly when they arrive. Hot foods should be served hot and cold foods served cold. Serving promptly maintains temperature and reduces the risk of foodborne infection. Food is more acceptable if the proper temperature is maintained.

Some residents wait in the dining room for a long time before meals are served. This is fine if the residents choose to do so, but they should not be required to wait for prolonged periods. Some facilities provide music, exercise, current events discussions, or activities to help the residents pass the time. This turns a boring wait into an enjoyable, stimulating activity.

Follow your facility's policies for preparing residents and the environment for meals. Some facilities require removal of laundry hampers and housekeeping carts from hallways before tray carts are delivered. Some residents must be prepared by covering with a clothing protector (Figure 7-1). Avoid calling a clothing protector a bib, which is a demeaning term to most adults. Some residents have medical conditions that cause them to be messy eaters. They may prefer to cover their clothing with an attractive hospital gown or poncho top, which is removed after meals. Many facilities have wet wipes available in or near the dining area so residents can wipe their faces and hands if they wish. Warm, packaged bathing products are appreciated and enjoyed by the residents (Figure 7-2 A & B).

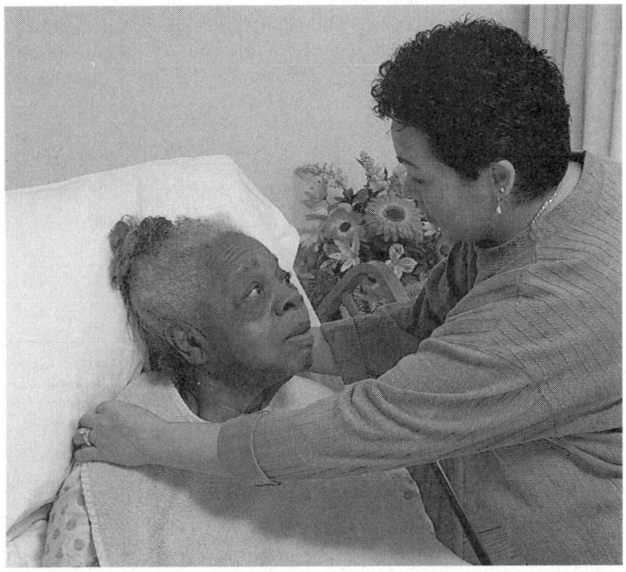

FIGURE 7-1
An adult clothing protector. Avoid referring to this garment as a bib.

Guidelines for Preparing for Meals

- Make the environment as pleasant as possible. Tables should be clean and ready, trash picked up, and the floor clear.
- Provide supplies for residents to wash their hands, if needed or desired.
- Be sure residents have dentures, glasses, and hearing aid, if used.
- Monitor the residents' positions and distance from the food and make necessary adjustments, if necessary.
- Apply a clothing protector, if used by the resident.

Positioning Residents for Meals

Proper positioning is important when seating residents at dining tables. Food is not swallowed or digested if the resident is not upright. Poor posture increases the

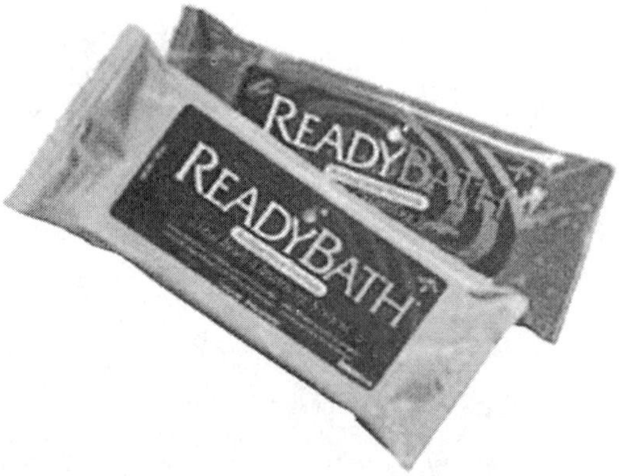

FIGURE 7-2A
Assist residents with washing hands and faces before and after meals. (Courtesy of Medline Industries, Inc. (800) MEDLINE.)

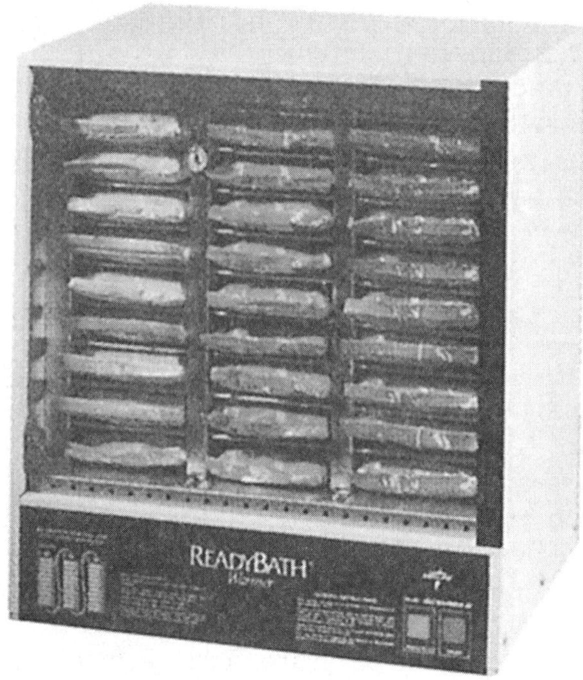

FIGURE 7-2B
Warm washcloths or disposable wipes are very refreshing. The microwave may cause hot spots. For safety, warm the bag bath products in the product warmer. (Courtesy of Medline Industries, Inc. (800) MEDLINE.)

risk of choking. Many facilities seat residents in regular dining chairs with arms at mealtime, rather than in wheelchairs. Some facilities have a "walk and dine" program in which wheelchairs are parked at the dining room door, and residents are assisted to walk to their tables. The care plan and the resident's medical condition will identify special positioning needs. Usually, residents should:

- Sit with the torso upright.
  - feet supported on footrests or the floor; they must never dangle
  - hips bent as closely to a 90-degree angle as possible
  - knees and ankles positioned at 90-degree angles
  - head forward with the chin down slightly
- Be close enough to the table that he or she does not have to stretch and reach to eat.
  - Residents should not have to extend their arms more than 10 to 12 inches to reach the food.
- Sit at a table that is not too high or too low.
  - Position residents so the elbows are below the hands when eating.
  - The elbows should be down. They should not be in the air when the resident reaches for food or when the resident is eating.
  - If the resident is too low, he or she must reach up to eat. Reaching up strains the shoulder and arm muscles and increases fatigue. Residents may become too tired to finish the meal.
- Make sure the resident's head is upright. If the head is tipped too far back, food may enter the airway. If the head is tipped too far forward, the resident may have difficulty breathing and swallowing.

Choking, aspiration, indigestion, and heartburn may result if the resident is not positioned properly for meals. If the resident has to work to eat, she or he may not eat as well. Mealtime will become a chore instead of a pleasure. A regular chair is

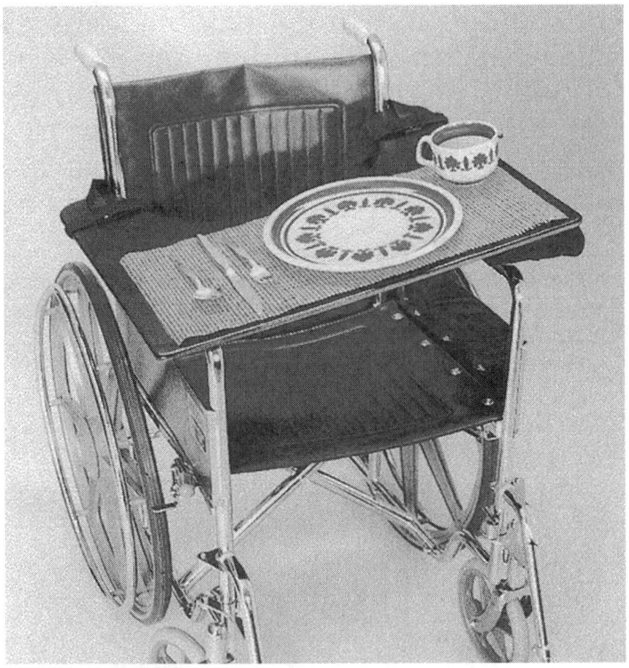

FIGURE 7-3
Some residents cannot reach their food when seated in a wheelchair at the table. Grouping residents in wheelchairs with removable trays provides the social atmosphere of mealtime, and makes it easier to eat. Adding gripper or another nonslip matting to the tray keeps dishes from sliding. (Courtesy of Skil-Care Corporation, Yonkers, NY (800) 431-2972.)

probably better at mealtime than a wheelchair. Wheelchair arms may not fit under the table and will increase the distance that the resident has to stretch. For residents in wheelchairs, a tray with Velcro fasteners (Figure 7-3) may make eating easier. Position the wheelchair next to the table to keep the resident from becoming isolated. If this is not possible, try grouping three or four residents with trays in a circle. This will provide the socialization and companionship they would have at a table.

SERVING MEALS

Food is served on trays in most facilities, although some have buffet lines and family-style meals. A few have selective menus. Trays are commonly delivered in carts. Serve trays promptly. Each tray will have a plastic **diet card** or paper printed on a computer that lists the resident's name, room number, and type of diet. Food allergies, preferences, dislikes, and adaptive devices used by the resident may also be listed.

Guidelines for Serving Meals

- Plan and organize your time so you are available to pass trays as soon as the food cart arrives.
- Wash your hands.
- Serve one table at a time. Residents should not have to watch their table mates eat while they are waiting for their own food. If possible, serve slow eaters first.
- If a closed cart is used, shut the door to the food cart as soon as you remove each tray. This helps maintain food temperature and prevents contamination.
- Check the diet card against the items on the tray for accuracy.
- Replace missing items, if needed.
- Keep food covered during transportation to maintain temperature and prevent contamination.
- Take the tray to the table and identify the resident.
- Remove food and place it on the table in front of the resident, if this is your facility's policy. If not, place the tray in front of the resident.
- Prepare the meal, if necessary, by removing covers, packages, and wrappers, such as foil and plastic; peeling food such as fruit; opening milk and yogurt cartons; providing straws; cutting meat; buttering bread; stirring sugar or lemon into beverages, if needed; and putting condiments on food.
- Position the plate with the main course closest to the resident.
- Assist the resident with the napkin.

- Provide adaptive eating devices, if used.
- Feed the resident, if necessary.
- Leave trays on the food cart until you are ready to feed residents. Do not put a tray in front of a resident who must be spoon-fed until you are available to assist with the meal.
- Serve all clean trays before returning used trays to the food cart. Do not return used trays if uneaten food remains on the cart.
- If you stop serving trays to assist a resident physically, wash your hands (or use alcohol hand cleaner) before continuing.

Make sure that residents have condiments and other seasonings of choice. After all trays are served, check on residents. Offer to replace or reheat food that has become cold. Honor resident requests for substitutes and extra portions, if allowed. Always offer beverage refills.

Liquids. Dehydration is a common problem in elderly persons, both in facilities and in the community. Mealtime is an excellent time to encourage liquids. Some facilities provide a glass of ice water on food trays. Many confused residents will drink whatever liquids are placed in front of them. Offer residents a second cup of coffee (or a beverage of choice) during or after meals. Long-term care residents will appreciate this gesture and benefit from the fluid intake. Making mealtime special will pay off in resident satisfaction, quality of life, and prevention of weight loss, malnutrition, and dehydration.

Food substitutes. Facilities prepare a substitute for the meat and vegetable at each meal. If the resident refuses an item, or eats less than 50% to 75% of these foods, a substitute should be offered. There is no requirement to substitute desserts or breads, but these may be provided, if permitted on the diet. Do not offer liquid commercial nutritional supplements as meal substitutes. Supplements must be medically prescribed and require a physician order. They are usually high in carbohydrates, but may not contain adequate protein. They contain sugar, which can be harmful to diabetics and those on special diets.

Guidelines for Assisting in the Dining Room

- Be aware of residents' self-feeding ability and changes in eating patterns. You will be feeding residents who are medically stable. Report observations and changes in residents' conditions and appetites to the nurse.
- Honor food preferences, likes, and dislikes.
- Offer a variety of foods and beverages. Always offer refills on beverages.
- Help residents who are having trouble feeding themselves.
- Notify the nurse if a resident has new problems with feeding, eating, or using utensils.
- Inform the nurse if a resident's alertness, responsiveness, ability to swallow, or positioning interferes with the ability to safely chew and swallow food.
- Prompt and encourage residents to eat.
- Allow enough time for residents to finish eating; avoid rushing them.
- If you are physically assisting more than one resident, wash your hands (or use an alcohol hand cleaner) before moving to the next resident.
- If a resident's appetite decreases, or he or she seems sad, ask if you can help. Inform the nurse.
- Inform the nurse if residents have complaints that you cannot resolve. If residents complain about food,

obtain objective information, such as "food is cold" or "food is too tough to chew."

- Use common sense and do your best to make mealtime satisfying.
- Monitor the floor. Food and beverages are slippery, and could cause ambulatory residents and staff to fall. Clean up spills promptly.
- Always wash your hands (or use an alcohol hand cleaner) when you have finished feeding residents, before leaving the dining area.
- Accurately record the residents' intake at each meal.

Socialization

Eating is a social time, and food satisfies emotional needs for many individuals. Think about it. Some people are uncomfortable going to a restaurant alone. We usually eat meals with one or more companions. Food choices and routines are affected by ethnicity, culture, and religion. Many family gatherings, social activities, and events revolve around food. Socialization is an important part of meal service. Most residents in long-term care facilities eat in community dining rooms. They look forward to meals. People eat better when they are in groups. Residents should be seated with others with whom they can socialize. Avoid positioning them so they are looking out a window or at a wall. Speak with residents when passing trays and assisting with meals. Stimulate resident socialization by using the meal as a topic of conversation. Residents may also enjoy discussing their interests, hobbies, or families. Encourage residents to participate by asking questions. To start a conversation:

- Identify the food. Discuss the flavor and texture.
- Discuss cooking or food preparation. Ask residents about how they formerly prepared and served this type of food. Ask how they like the food seasoned.
- Talk about your favorite foods. Ask residents about their favorites.

ASSISTING RESIDENTS WITH FEEDING

Some residents are not able to eat by themselves and must be fed. They may feel embarrassed and childish. Be sensitive to the residents' feelings.

Guidelines for Feeding Residents

- Wash your hands (or use an alcohol hand cleaner) before beginning.
- Sit at or below the resident's eye level, if possible. This is less intimidating than standing over the resident. It also prevents the resident from choking, which could be caused by bending the head back and looking up at you.
- Check the food temperature before feeding. Place a drop of hot food on your wrist to be sure it is not too hot.
- If the food is too hot, wait a few minutes before serving the tray. Never blow on or fan the food. Allow it to cool on its own. Recheck the temperature before serving.
- Tell the resident what is on the tray. Ask what the resident would like to eat first. For residents who regularly request dessert first, say, "Do you want to start with the casserole?"
- Never mix food items together, unless requested by the resident. Feed each food item separately.
- Sometimes residents cannot handle utensils, but can eat finger foods, such as bread, crackers, or cookies. Encourage them to do this, if able.

- Offer liquids at intervals. Using a straw will make it easier for residents to drink.
- Make pleasant conversation while feeding the resident. Listen to what the resident says. Avoid making conversation if the resident coughs or has difficulty swallowing. Responding to conversation may cause accidental choking.
- Treat the resident with respect and kindness.
- Anticipate needs.
- Avoid rushing the resident.
- Be emotionally sensitive to residents' needs. Focus on residents when feeding. Avoid having conversations with other staff in the room. If you converse with other staff members while feeding, include residents in the conversation.
- If a resident cannot stay awake during the meal, or if he or she repeatedly coughs, gags, or chokes, stop feeding and request a nursing assessment.
- Wash your hands (or use an alcohol hand cleaner) after removing a food tray, before assisting other residents.

Procedure 5—Feeding the Dependent Resident

1. Wash your hands (or use an alcohol hand cleaner).
2. Prepare the resident and obtain the tray.
3. Place the tray on the table and sit at or below the resident's eye level. Sit on the resident's right if you are right-handed, or the left if you are left-handed.
4. Offer the resident water or a cool liquid to moisten the mouth and throat and test ability to swallow.
   - Follow the care plan for giving liquids. Use a straw, if the resident is able.
   - Some residents can drink directly from a small paper cup that you bend and conform to the resident's mouth. Check with the nurse before offering a beverage in a styrofoam cup. Residents occasionally bite the cup and swallow the foam.
5. Inform the resident what is on the tray and ask what he or she would like to eat first.
6. Fill the fork or spoon half full.
   - If the resident has not requested a specific food item, inform him or her what you are offering first.
   - Using the spoon, apply gentle downward pressure on the lips or tip of the tongue if the resident does not respond by opening the mouth.
   - If the resident has had a stroke, place food in the unaffected side of the mouth.
7. Alternate liquids and solids. The resident may want a drink after every third or fourth spoonful of food.
   - Pace the feeding to allow the resident time to chew and swallow safely.
8. Converse with the resident during the meal. Tell him what you are giving him.
9. Wipe the resident's mouth and hands as often as necessary.
10. Remove the tray when the resident is finished.
11. Wash the resident's hands and face, if necessary.
12. Remove the clothing protector.
13. Remove food from the clothing or wheelchair, if necessary.
14. Remove the tray.
15. Wash your hands (or use an alcohol hand cleaner).

16. Record the resident's appetite and fluid intake according to facility policy.

Special Problems

Some residents have medical problems that interfere with their ability to eat. Become familiar with, and follow the feeding care plan for these individuals. Suggestions for assisting residents with common problems are listed below.

Cognitive impairment. Residents with cognitive impairment are easily distracted and may not eat well. They are busy monitoring the activity in the room instead of eating. Approaches that may help them are:

- Seat residents in a quiet area.
- Reduce activity near the table as much as possible.
- Do not position their chairs facing the center of the room.
- A corner of the dining room may be screened off for special needs residents, or they may be served in a different area entirely. Some facilities serve meals in two shifts.
- Small, frequent meals may work better than larger ones.
- Avoid long waiting times. Escort the resident to the table and serve immediately.
- If the resident is not interested in eating, begin with a small amount of cold, slightly thick liquid or several small spoons of sherbet to stimulate swallowing.
- Bowls may work better than plates.
- Cups with large handles work well.
- Spoons may be better than forks.
- Offer one food item at a time.
- Persuade the resident to take a bite of each food.
- Compliment the resident for making an effort.

Vision impairment. Some residents have difficulty eating or poor appetite because of vision problems. They do not eat their meals because they cannot see them. Some are fed by staff because their visual problem is unrecognized and uncorrected. Getting them glasses may enable them to feed themselves. Other residents may need their prescription glasses changed. Some residents who have had strokes have a condition called **hemianopsia**. They have blindness in half the visual field. If you notice a resident has eaten the food on only one side of the plate or tray, turn it around. He or she may not be able to see the food on both sides of the tray. Suspect vision problems if the resident:

- tries to pick up food several times before finally scooping it up
- cannot move the utensil to the mouth without spilling (This does not apply to residents with tremors and neurological problems.)
- eventually becomes frustrated and stops eating

If you believe a visual problem is interfering with the resident's ability to eat, inform the nurse.

Legal blindness. People who are legally blind can usually feed themselves. They memorize the location of items. Moving things could result in accidents, injuries, or frustration because the resident is unable to find a needed item. When serving a meal tray to a visually impaired or blind resident, describe the location of food items compared with a clock (Figure 7-4). Say, "The bread is at 10:00, meat loaf is at 6:00, and the milk is at 2:00." Identify the items on the tray clearly. Instead of saying, "The casserole is at 6:00," describe what is in the casserole, such as beef, mushrooms, and beans. Instead of saying, "dessert," identify the item, such as "apple pie." Inform the resident if you

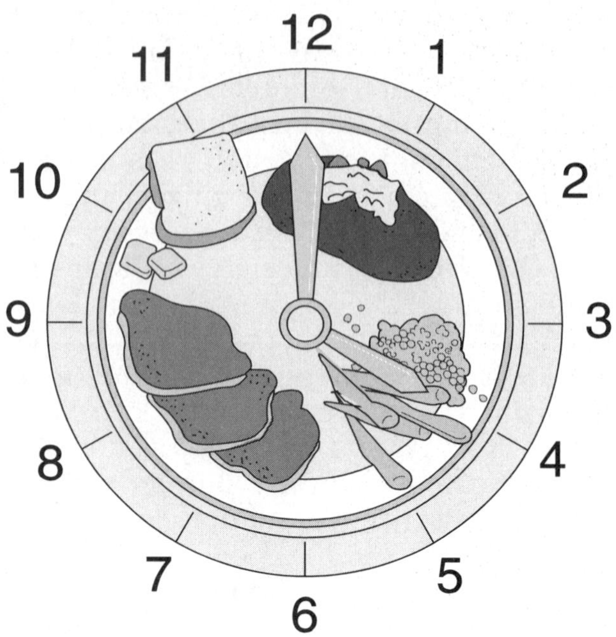

FIGURE 7-4
When serving a tray to a resident with visual impairment, describe the arrangement of the food compared with the face of a clock.

have buttered the bread, put a straw in (or poured) the milk, or seasoned any of the items on the tray. For example, "You asked for vinegar on your spinach, so I put it in a separate bowl at 4:00 to keep the vinegar from running into your other food." The resident uses your words in place of eyes, so painting a specific verbal picture will help him or her immensely.

Resident bites utensils. Avoid using plastic utensils, which may injure the resident. Ask the resident to open the mouth. Wait until he or she does so, or until the muscles relax. Never try to force the utensil out of the mouth.

Wandering. Some residents wander constantly, including during mealtimes. The wandering consumes extra calories. This places them at high risk for weight loss. Since staff are often busy immediately before, during, and after meals, this is an opportune time for wanderers to exit the facility. In fact, they are often discovered missing when staff attempts to serve their meal tray. Because of this, residents who wander need close supervision before, during, and after meals. Inform the nurse immediately if a resident is missing. If the noise and stimulation in the dining area seem to overwhelm the resident, she or he may do better eating in a quiet, supervised area.

Residents who wander often present challenges at mealtime, because they may not sit long enough to eat. Techniques for assisting this resident include:

- Serve the resident promptly. Do not make her wait.
- If the resident leaves the table, try to coax her back. Approach from the front, then walk with the resident by falling in step at her side. Walk with her and circle back in.
- Try to distract her with food, drink, or conversation.
- Walk with the resident and give her finger foods, such as a sandwich, if necessary.
- Provide finger foods between meals.

Tremors. Some residents have neurologic problems and chronic conditions that cause shaking and tremors. Hand and arm tremors cause food to spill before reaching the mouth. This is upsetting to the resident, and reduces the intake of needed nutrients. Some residents wear weighted hand splints (Figure 7-5) to reduce the tremors, enabling them to eat. Other approaches to use are:

- Make sure the resident is upright and well supported in the chair.
- Position the resident as close to the plate as possible.
- Support the forearms and elbows on the table or the arms of the chair.
- Provide foods that are easy to handle. For example, creamed corn is easier to eat than whole kernel corn.

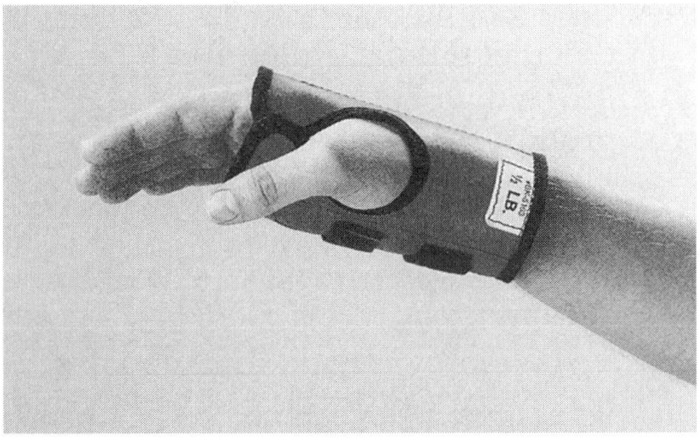

FIGURE 7-5
Weighted hand splints reduce the tremors of multiple sclerosis, Parkinson's disease, and other neurologic conditions. This enables the resident to feed herself with less spilling. (Courtesy of Sammons Preston, Inc. Reprinted with permission.)

- Be patient and supportive.
- Provide assistive devices.
- If the resident is embarrassed or self-conscious, consider other seating arrangements. If possible, seat the resident with an easy-going, compassionate resident. Avoid isolating the resident.

Paralysis and limited movement. The ability to move voluntarily is a good predictor of dependency. Residents with movement in one arm can often feed themselves after the tray is prepared. Assistive devices may increase eating independence. Special cups, dishes, utensils, or placemats enable residents to feed themselves with dignity.

Sensory disorders. The sensory response to food is complicated. The brain coordinates signals of smell and taste with sight, temperature, and texture. Sensory disorders have many causes, including normal aging, various diseases, lack of certain vitamins and minerals, certain medications, cigarette smoking, and wearing dentures. Sensory problems are difficult to overcome. Sensory problems may affect:

- temperature
- smell
- taste
- hearing and vision
- touch
- texture

The presentation and attractiveness of food are especially important for residents whose smell, taste, and texture sensations are impaired. They may not be able to smell the food. Taste and texture sensations may be altered. Always check food temperature. This is particularly important with hot foods. All residents are at risk of burns if food is too hot. Residents with abnormal temperature sensations are at greater risk than others. The facility dietitian and occupational, physical, and speech therapists will work with residents to help resolve sensory problems.

Resident wants dessert first. Provide a nutritious alternative to dessert, such as fruit. Then suggest the resident try the meat or another specific food item on the tray.

Resident will not open mouth. Ask the resident to open the mouth. If this does not work, place some food on the spoon and touch the resident's lips with it. Yawn. If you yawn, the resident may yawn also. However, you must have good timing. Avoid slipping food into the mouth when the resident is inhaling.

Resident refuses to eat. Try to determine why the resident will not eat and correct the problem. Ask the resident. Encourage the resident to eat by setting a goal. Offer foods the resident likes. Notify the nurse of the refusal.

Resident holds food in mouth or pockets in cheek. Gently pushing on the front of the tongue when removing the spoon will trigger swallowing. Other useful approaches are:

- Tell the resident to chew and/or swallow.
- Offer a sip of liquid.
- Touch the top of the head gently.
- Touch the cheek and tell the resident to use the tongue to get the food.
- Check the mouth to make sure it is empty before giving more food, and also at the end of the meal.

Resident plays with food. Provide one item at a time. Cue the resident and encourage her or him to eat. Provide cups with lids and straws.

MAINTAINING INDEPENDENCE

There is a common expression, "If you don't use it, you lose it." This is particularly true of self-care tasks. If a resident does not use life care skills, he or she will eventually lose the ability to do them. Because of this, you are not doing residents a favor by performing tasks that they can do for themselves. Being independent helps residents feel good about themselves. The ability to choose food and eat independently affects residents' appetites. Inability to feed oneself is associated with a higher death rate. Do not underestimate confused residents' ability for self-care. Test their ability. Provide support and direction, if needed. Eating part of a meal independently is better than not at all. You may be surprised to find that some residents can do a great deal by themselves. Enabling and encouraging residents to eat independently will help maintain their ability.

Guidelines for Encouraging and Maintaining Mealtime Independence

- Follow the resident's feeding care plan.
- Set up (provide and prepare) needed materials.
- Give simple instructions and demonstrations, if necessary.
- Provide verbal cues (hints) to prompt the resident, if necessary.
- Repeat directions and hints, if necessary.
- Provide support, encouragement, and praise.
- Use hand-over-hand technique, if necessary. Cover the resident's hand with your hand, then guide the hand to the mouth.
- Be patient. Allow as much time as necessary.
- If the resident is unable to finish, allow her to do all she can, then offer to feed her the rest.
- If the resident cannot use utensils, have him hold and eat finger foods.
- Always stress the resident's ability, not the disability. For example, avoid saying, "You *cannot use* your right hand to pick up your cookie." Instead say, "You *can use* your left hand to eat your cookie."
- Reheat food if it becomes cold.
- If the resident is relearning a skill, work on one step at a time. When the resident masters one step, move to the next.
- Remember that the resident's progress may be inconsistent from day to day. Encourage the resident.
- Praise the resident for what she or he was able to do.
- Avoid making the resident feel like a failure.

Following the Care Plan for Encouraging Mealtime Independence

You will see several different techniques for assisting residents with meals listed on the care plans. The most common approaches are:

- **Set up** means preparing the resident, food tray, plate, adaptive equipment, and other supplies.
- **Verbal cues** are hints that prompt the resident to do something. A cue is a brief, clear, and concise direction. You may need to repeat each cue several times.
- **Demonstration** is showing the resident what you want him or her to do. Show the resident how to do the skill. Simultaneously, give simple verbal directions. You will find methods of demonstration that work best for each resident. Some residents will require a demonstration of each step of the procedure. Others will be able to remember and follow more complete directions.
- **Hand-over-hand technique** is placing your hand over the resident's hand and guiding him or her to perform the desired action.

Residents with these care plan approaches may also receive finger food snacks during the day, such as cookies or popsicles. The hand-to-mouth motion for eating finger food is the same motion used for feeding. These approaches will gradually help the resident gain independence, so your assistance should fade out over time. Be patient, positive, and persistent. This could take weeks or months, but relearning this basic task is possible for many residents.

Instructions, Verbal Cues, and Commands

The resident must know what to do and what is expected. To succeed, he or she must make an effort. Fortunately, the resident will get hungry, so food is a good incentive. If the resident does not respond to verbal cues, move to hand-over-hand technique. Spoon-feeding is the last resort, not the initial response. Exhaust your options before spoon-feeding. Feeding the resident immediately may worsen dependence. Give the resident the opportunity to feed himself first. After exhausting the care plan approaches, finish feeding him, if necessary. Praise him for his efforts.

Verbal cues are things upon which the resident must act. To be effective, they must be properly timed. Time each cue to occur in sequence at the proper time. Repeat the steps as often as necessary to prompt the resident to do the task. Some residents will require a cue for each step of the meal. This takes patience and time.

General Guidelines for Verbal Cues

- Explain what you want the resident to do in simple terms.
- Allow the resident to ask questions, if able.
- Ask the resident if he or she understands. If the resident responds, this gives you an idea of the resident's understanding.
- Demonstrate the task several times, if necessary. People remember more of what they see than what they hear.
- Inform the resident that you will help and provide support.
- Make sure the resident can hear you.
- Speak slowly, clearly, and distinctly. Use simple terms. Avoid long, complicated directions.
- Vary your tone of voice, if necessary. For example, a sharp, quick command such as "Watch out!" will cause the resident to react quickly. He or she will respond more slowly to a soft, drawn-out command.
- Give simple, direct cues, one at a time. Specify the action required. For example, you will say:
  - "Pick up the spoon."
  - "Put the spoon in the applesauce."
  - "Scoop the applesauce onto the spoon."

- "Put the spoon in your mouth."
- "Chew."
- "Swallow."
- "Good!" or "Great!"
- "Take the spoon out of your mouth."
- Praise the resident for his or her accomplishment.
- Over time, fade out the prompting to help the resident gain independence.
- If the resident does not respond, demonstrate again, if necessary.
- If the resident still does not respond, progress to hand-over-hand technique.

Hand-Over-Hand Technique

If verbal cues are ineffective, use hand-over-hand technique to help the resident begin the task (Figure 7-6).

Guidelines for Hand-Over-Hand Technique

(These guidelines use a spoon as an example, but the name of any other utensil may be substituted for the word "spoon.")

- Tell the resident what you are doing. Use simple, direct terms.
- Demonstrate what you want the resident to do.
- Place the spoon in the resident's hand.
- Place your hand over the resident's hand.
- Guide the resident's hand to the plate.
- Guide the resident to fill the spoon.
- Remove your hand and see if the resident completes the step after getting started. If not, move to the next step.
- Guide the resident's hand back to his or her mouth.

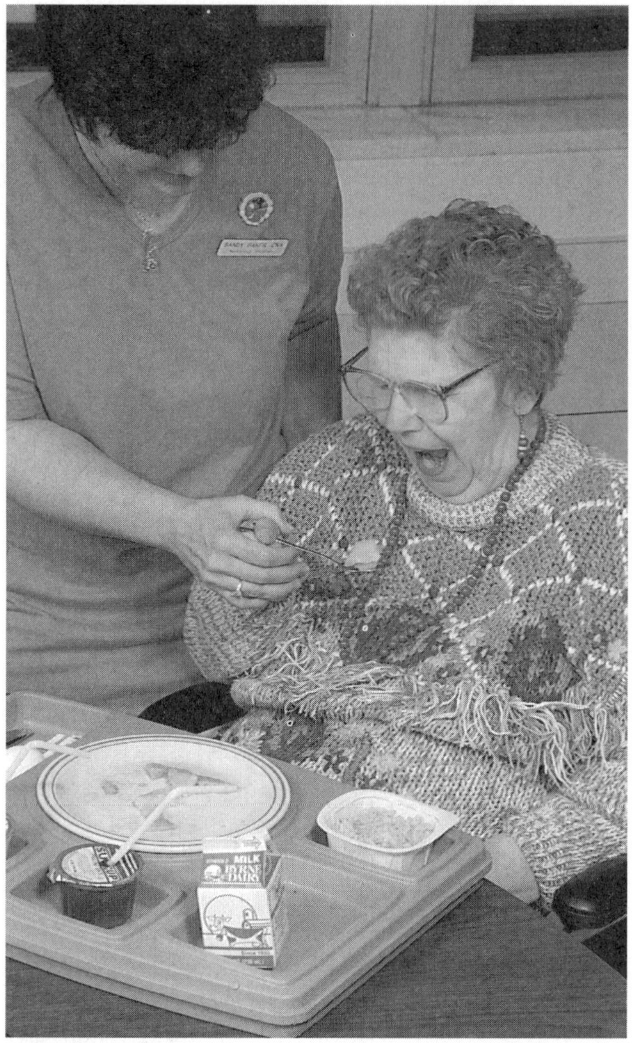

FIGURE 7-6
Use hand-over-hand technique if the resident does not respond to verbal cues.

- Gently touch the lips with the spoon, or instruct the resident to open his or her mouth.
- Repeat these steps again. Try to fade out by encouraging the resident to bring the filled spoon to his or her mouth. Support the wrist or forearm, if necessary.
- Repeat again. Use hand-over-hand technique to fill the spoon. Encourage the resident to direct the spoon to the mouth.

- Encourage the resident to try again after using hand-over-hand technique once or twice.
- Gradually reduce the physical assistance. This may take days or weeks. Be positive and persistent. Try to get the resident to the point where he or she responds to verbal cues 100% of the time.
- Avoid rushing the resident. Reheat the food, or get fresh food, if necessary. The resident will probably not eat well if the hot foods are cold and cold foods are warm.
- Continue using a combination of verbal cues and hand-over-hand technique.
- Praise the resident for his or her accomplishment.

ADAPTIVE DEVICES FOR EATING

Some residents have poor intake because they have difficulty feeding themselves. Others eat their food, but struggle with utensils because of physical problems or spilling. The therapist or restorative nurse will evaluate these residents for adaptive eating devices. Using adaptive devices will make eating or drinking easier. Notify the nurse if you feel a resident would benefit from an adaptive eating device.

Adaptive devices are equipment and utensils used to assist residents to perform everyday tasks. The devices change the way the task is done, enabling the resident to be more independent. Some adaptive devices are simple things that can be made by staff. For example, a bicycle hand grip may be attached to a spoon, so it is easier for the resident to hold. The facility must make sure the device can be thoroughly washed and sanitized. Because of this, many facilities purchase commercial devices. Many different devices are available. The occupational therapist or restorative nurse will have a catalog of these items. Look through it. You may be surprised at the diversity of products available. Using adaptive devices improves self-esteem. The resident can complete the task according to his or her own schedule, not someone else's.

The most common adaptive devices are used for feeding. If you are responsible for obtaining these devices, do so before the meal is served so the resident does not have to wait to eat. Many facilities list them on the diet card and the dietary department provides them with the tray. Common devices are found in Box 7-1.

When an adaptive device is first introduced, licensed personnel may work with the resident. They will teach the resident how to use the device. However, learning takes time. You may be asked to continue working with the resident until he or she masters it. Using hand-over-hand technique is helpful when a resident is learning to use utensils. When a utensil is introduced in this manner, the resident quickly sees that the device will make eating easier. However, he or she may need daily assistance, cues, and practice until mastering the device. Provide support and encouragement. Inform the nurse if a resident experiences a problem or if you feel a modification or change is needed.

Become familiar with the devices used in your facility, and learn how to use them. In some facilities, restorative nursing personnel work with residents using these devices. However, you must be able to identify the device and make sure it is clean and available when you serve meal trays.

AFTER MEALS

Check trays for personal items, such as dentures, glasses, or hearing aids. Residents commonly wrap these items in napkins and set them on trays. They are expensive and will not survive a trip through the dishwasher.

BOX 7-1

- *Plate guards* (Figure 7-7A) and *plates with built-up edges* (Figure 7-7B and 7-7C) are useful to keep the resident from pushing food off the plate when trying to scoop the food onto a utensil. The resident can also use one hand to hold a *piece of bread* on the plate. He or she can scoop food onto the utensil by pushing against the bread.
- *Built-up handles* on silverware (Figure 7-7D) make the utensil easier to grip. The rings adjust for resident comfort and function.
- Cutlery that is *angled* (Figure 7-7E) prevents spilling and makes self-feeding easier. *Utensils that swivel* are used to keep food from falling off the utensil for residents with tremors or weakness.
- Residents who cannot grasp silverware at all may use *utensils with a clip, hand grip, or Velcro cuff* that wraps around the hand (Figure 7-7F).
- *Adaptive cups* (Figure 7-7G) have lids and spouts that dispense a controlled amount of beverage. This cup is sometimes used for thickened liquids. When the rubber ring is pushed, liquid is dispensed into the spout.
- *Cups with special hand grips* (Figure 7-7H) or *lids* (Figure 7-7I) enable residents to bring them to the mouth without spilling.
- The *straw holder* (Figure 7-7J) may be used to keep the straw from moving. An alternative to a straw holder is *taping the straw* to the side of the cup. *Cutting the straw* will keep the straw from moving and make it easier for weak residents to drink.
- *Nonslip matting* (Figure 7-7K). Nonslip matting, a gripper, or a *damp washcloth* will secure the plate. Some residents scoop food away from their bodies, causing the plate to slide to the center of the table. Resting the resident's elbow on a piece of gripper or foam helps decrease movement and tremors.

After meals, pick up trays and return them to the tray cart. Wait until all uneaten trays have been passed before returning used trays to the cart. Remove the residents' clothing protectors, and provide supplies for wiping faces and hands, if needed or desired. Make sure there is no food on the face, hands, or clothing. Wipe spilled food off the wheelchair, if necessary. After all residents are cared for, finish clearing tables and straightening the dining room, according to your job description.

Documentation

Facilities document and record the amount of food residents consume in the medical record. A clipboard is commonly used to record meal intake in the dining room. The information is later transferred to the resident's chart. Remember that documented information is confidential. Keep the information covered with a piece of paper when the clipboard is not in use.

Each facility has a method for recording meal intake. Many use fractions or record the percentage of the diet consumed (Figure 7-8). Some write "good," "fair," or "poor." Some facilities record the percentage of each food item. Know and follow your facility's policy. Notify the nurse if a resident eats less than 75% of the meal, or according to facility policy. Follow the nurses' instructions. Record the amount of liquid taken if the resident is on intake and output (Chapter 8). Examples of several additional meal intake recording systems are in Appendix A.

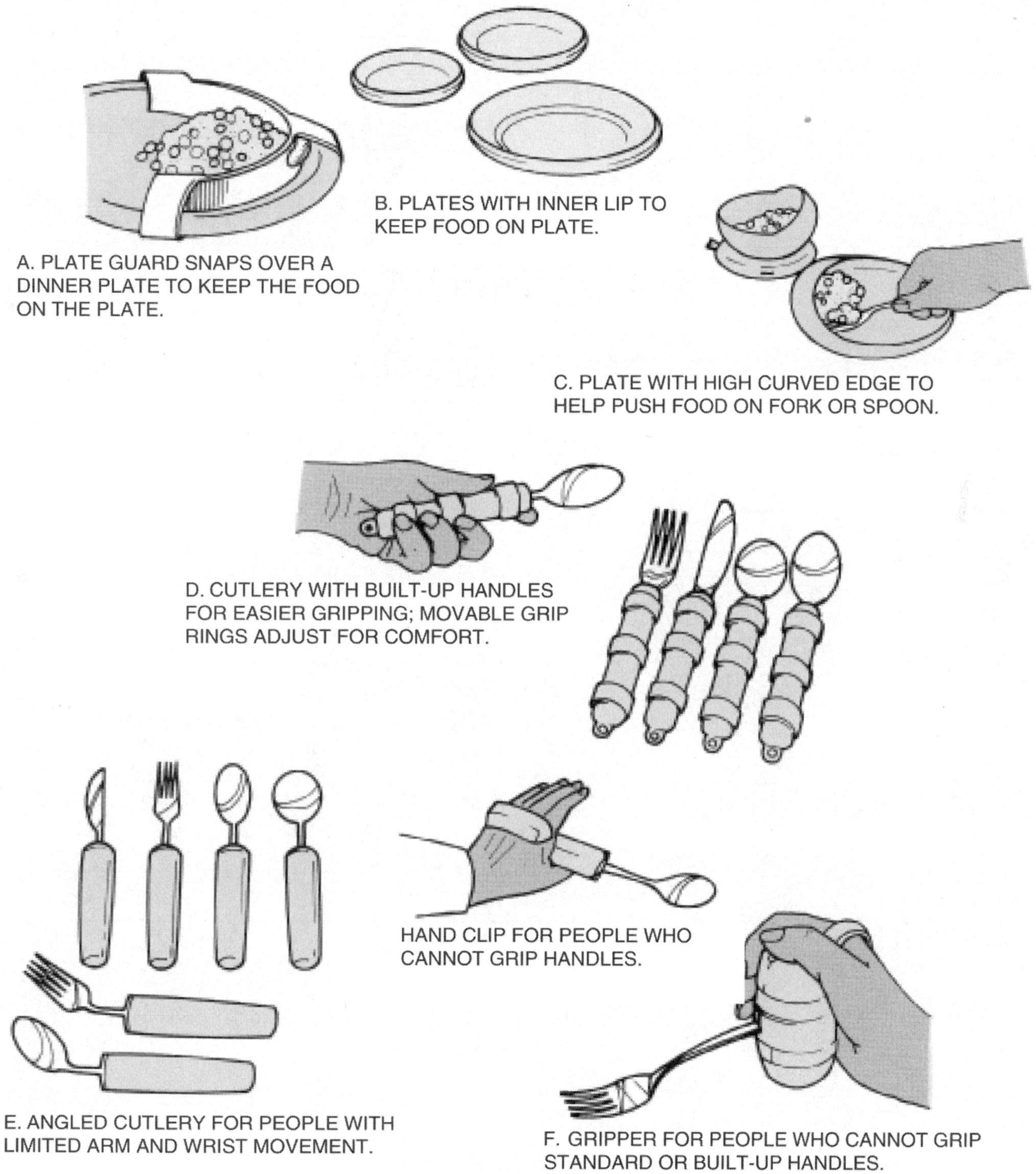

FIGURE 7-7A-F
Many types of adaptive utensils are available to meet individual needs and enable residents to feed themselves.

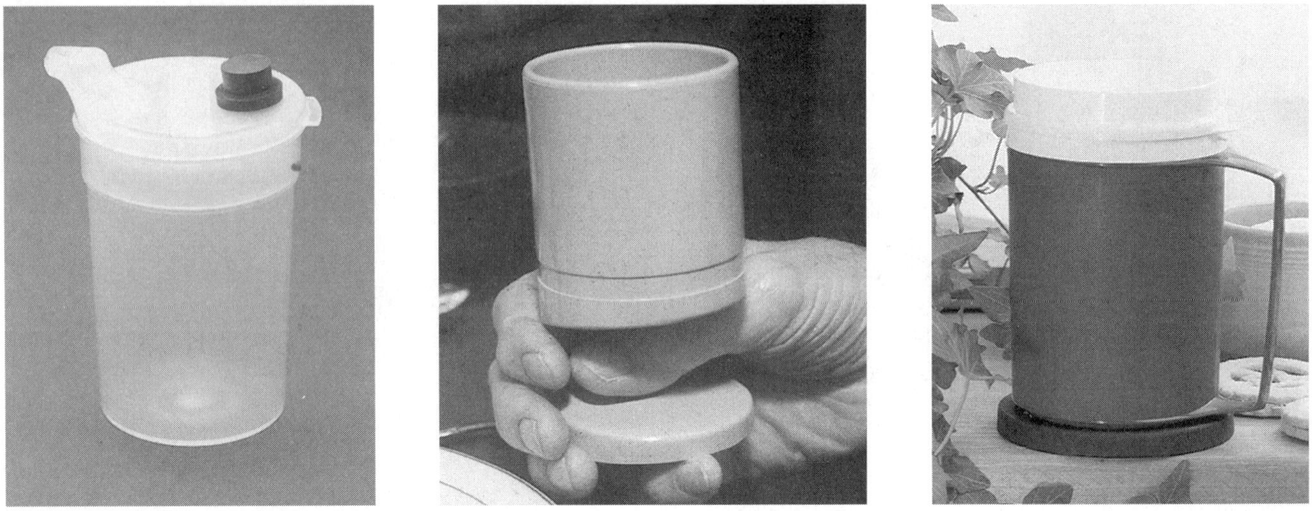

FIGURE 7-7G-I
Many special cups are available to meet the residents' needs.

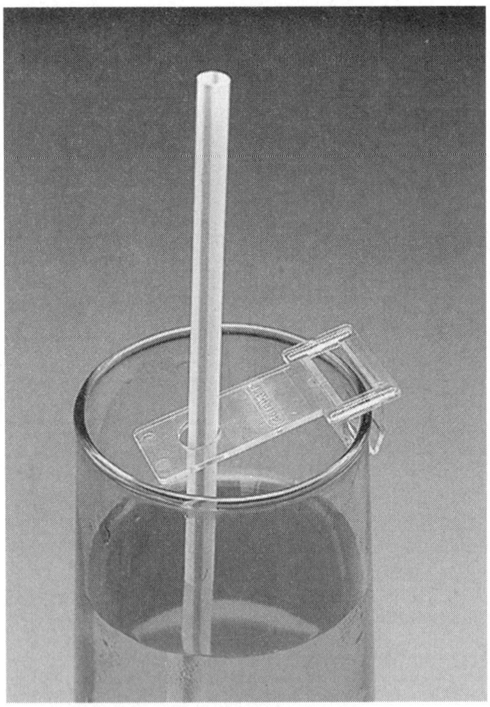

FIGURE 7-7J
The straw holder conveniently holds the straw so the resident will not have to chase it. (Courtesy of Maddak, Inc.).

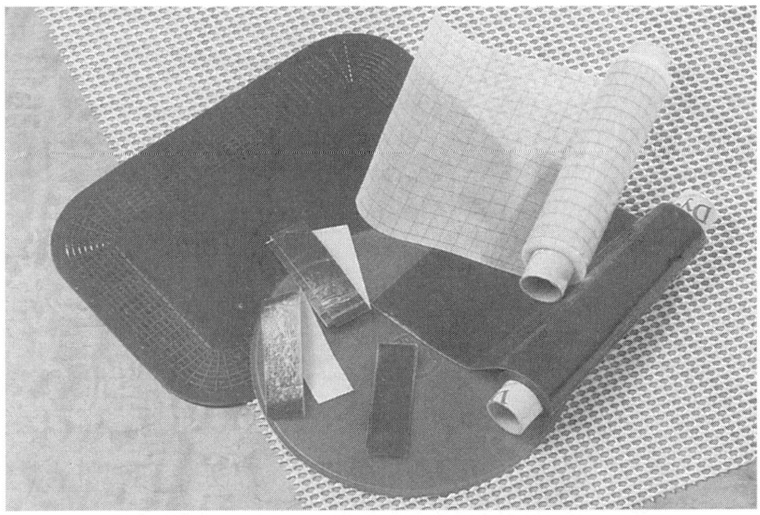

FIGURE 7-7K
Nonslip matting has hundreds of uses. Positioning it under a plate or the resident's arm will prevent slipping. The matting may be rinsed, air dried, and reused. It should not be used when wet. (Courtesy of Sammons Preston, Inc. Reprinted with permission.)

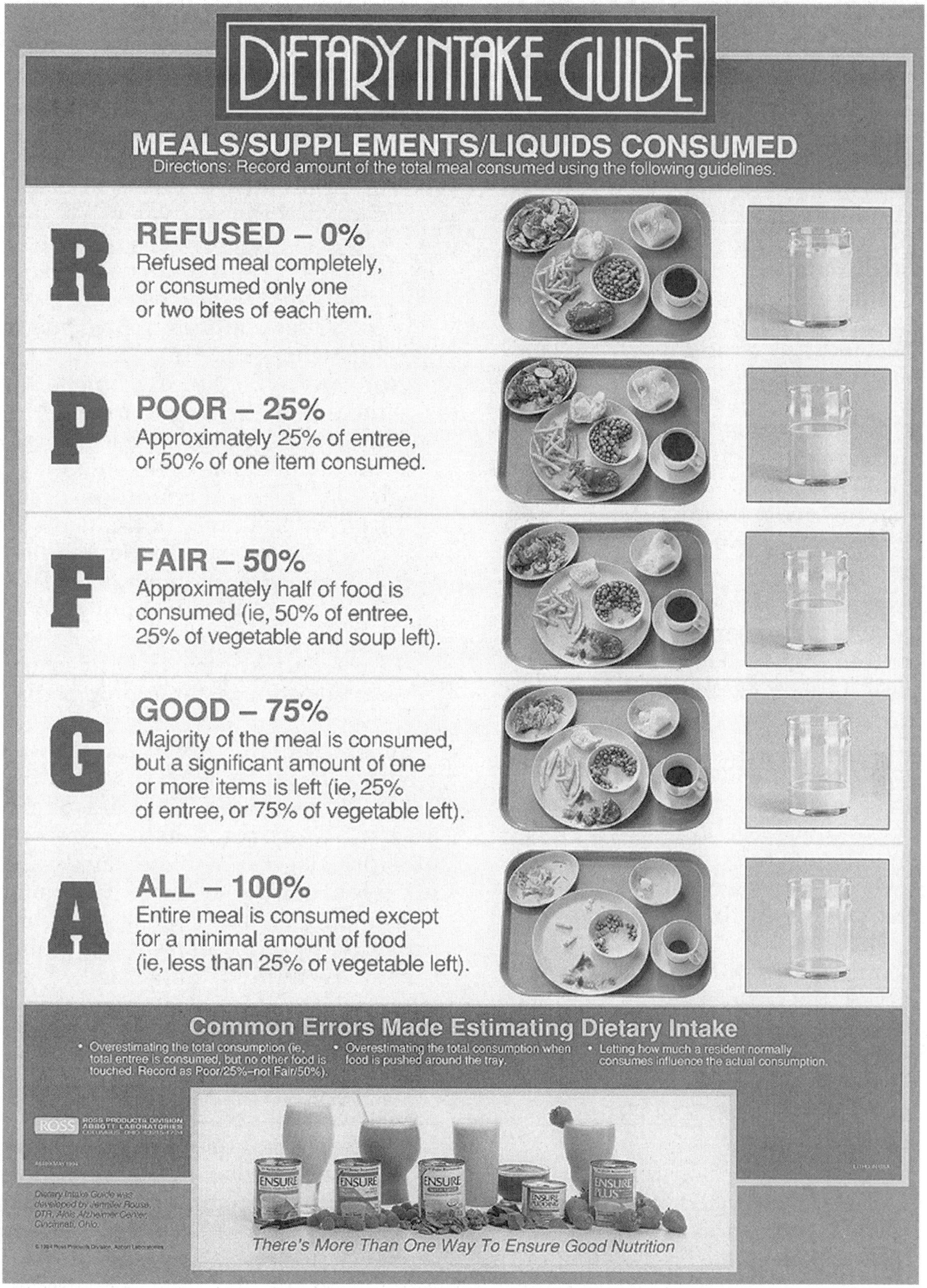

FIGURE 7-8
Accurate documentation of meal intake is an important responsibility. (Used with permission of Ross Products Division, Abbott Laboratories, Columbus, Ohio.)

SNACKS, NOURISHMENTS, AND SUPPLEMENTS

No uniform definitions are available for snacks, supplements, and nourishments. In fact, some dictionaries treat these items as synonyms. Because of the lack of uniform definitions, facilities have various individual definitions, policies, and procedures for their use. Become familiar with the definitions and policies used in your facility.

- **Snacks** are *light foods* that are *given to any resident* between meals and at bedtime, as permitted by diet order. A specific *physician order is not needed* unless the resident is on a restricted diet. Snacks include items such as graham crackers, fruit, and cookies.
- **Nourishments** are *more substantial* food items that are given to increase nutrient intake. They are commonly given to *selected residents* to prevent weight loss or increase weight. They are usually *planned and ordered by the facility dietitian* and include foods such as sandwiches, instant breakfast, milkshakes, pudding, whole milk, yogurt, cottage cheese, and ice cream. Nourishments are sometimes made from the previous day's leftovers. For example, if roast turkey dinner was served, the leftover turkey would be used to make turkey sandwiches or turkey salad for those residents receiving nourishments. Nourishments provide more nutrients than snacks.
- **Supplements** are usually *liquid nutritional products* that are ordered by the physician for *specific residents* to help them gain weight or to correct a specific medical problem. Supplements are given to make up for a deficiency, strengthen the whole body, or promote healing. Supplemental puddings are also available. These are largely high-calorie carbohydrate products. Most, but not all, contain approximately one calorie per milliliter (mL) of liquid. A milliliter is a form of liquid measure used in health care. It is the equivalent of one cubic centimeter (cc). (Most supplements come in 8 ounce containers. There are 30 mL per ounce, so one container contains approximately 240 calories.) Many different flavors are available. For example, eggnog flavor may be served over the Christmas holidays. Specialized supplements are available for certain medical conditions, such as diabetes, renal (kidney) disease, and pulmonary disease. Liquid nutritional supplements are filling. Because of this, they are served between meals and not with meals. In some facilities, only licensed nurses administer supplements.

Most residents prefer liquid supplements and nourishments served cold. If the beverage is warm, the resident may not accept it. Since some of these products are milk-based, serving them warm can be an infection control hazard. Supplements, nourishments, and snacks are usually provided by the dietary department and served by nursing personnel. They are labeled with the resident's name. If perishable items are provided, refrigerate them until they are served.

When serving supplements and nourishments, make sure the resident can consume the item independently. Do not set it down and walk away. Pour the beverage into a cup, if preferred by the resident. Provide a straw. If the resident cannot manage the product, assist him or her. Encourage the resident to drink it. You may have to spoon-feed the resident items such as pudding. Document the resident's food acceptance on the proper form. Record the amount of liquid if the resident is on intake and output. Inform the nurse if the resident expresses a preference or dislike for a certain product or flavor.

CHAPTER REVIEW

Multiple Choice

Select the one best answer.

1. Being dependent on others may cause feelings of:
   - **a.** satisfaction.
   - **b.** increased pleasure.
   - **c.** decreased self-esteem.
   - **d.** superiority.
2. When seating residents for meals:
   - **a.** Consider table height and distance from the table.
   - **b.** Always seat dependent residents in wheelchairs.
   - **c.** Elbow and shoulder positions are not important.
   - **d.** The forearms should rest on the table surface.
3. Long-term care facilities are required to provide substitutes for the:
   - **a.** bread and fruit.
   - **b.** meat and vegetable.
   - **c.** beverage and dessert.
   - **d.** milk and salad.
4. If the resident does not eat his or her meal:
   - **a.** Inform the nurse.
   - **b.** Offer a liquid nutritional supplement.
   - **c.** Assume the resident is not hungry.
   - **d.** Buy something from the vending machines.
5. If a resident does not respond to verbal cues to eat:
   - **a.** Report to the nurse.
   - **b.** Spoon-feed the resident.
   - **c.** Consult a nursing assistant.
   - **d.** Use hand-over-hand technique.
6. Mr. Healey began a feeding program three days ago. Today, he seems tired and is not responding to your verbal cues. Your next step is to:
   - **a.** Feed the resident.
   - **b.** Take his temperature.
   - **c.** Use hand-over-hand technique.
   - **d.** Notify the dietitian.
7. Guidelines for passing trays to residents include all of the following except:
   - **a.** handwashing and identifying the resident.
   - **b.** serving trays to residents who must be fed, then returning later to feed them.
   - **c.** checking the food on the tray against the diet on the diet card to see if it is allowed.
   - **d.** preparing the tray, as needed, and providing adaptive devices.
8. Check the temperature of hot food items by:
   - **a.** getting a glass thermometer from the nursing unit.
   - **b.** sticking your finger into each hot food item.
   - **c.** using the spoon to place a drop of food on your wrist.
   - **d.** touching the bottom of the plate with your elbow.
9. If you feel food is too hot to feed to a dependent resident, you should:
   - **a.** Return the food to the tray cart uneaten.
   - **b.** Blow on the food to cool it.
   - **c.** Put the food in the refrigerator.
   - **d.** Leave the food until it cools.
10. Which of the following is true?
    - **a.** Confused residents do not enjoy their food.
    - **b.** Satisfaction with food affects quality of life.
    - **c.** Give the residents supplements if they eat less than 50%.
    - **d.** Open the food cart door so food cools quickly.

UNIT 8

Hydration and Fluid Intake

OBJECTIVES

- Spell and define key terms.
- Briefly explain why water is needed, and why maintaining fluid balance is important.
- Give an overview of an elderly person's minimum daily fluid requirements.
- Define dehydration and list reasons that residents do not consume enough fluids each day.
- List risk factors for dehydration.
- Demonstrate accurate measurement of oral fluid intake.
- List the general rules for serving fresh drinking water.

FLUID BALANCE

Water is essential to life and health. Fluid fills space within and between body cells. Every cell, tissue, organ, and system in the body needs water to function properly. Water is an essential nutrient because the body requires more than it can produce. Water supplies and carries nutrients, transports wastes and toxins, and helps regulate body temperature. It has many other functions as well.

Water works with sodium, calcium, and other items to maintain fluid balance in the body, which is critical to good health. Major organ failure will occur if the balance of fluid and minerals is not maintained. We can survive for at least six weeks without food. However, we could not survive more than a week without water.

Dehydration

Most adults take in 2 to 3 quarts of liquid each day. Most of this is consumed in the form of liquid beverages and water. Some foods, fruits, and vegetables also provide water. On the average, facility residents need 1.5 to 2 quarts a day, or 1600 mL to 2000 mL. Some residents need more than this. The dietitian calculates the minimum daily fluid needs for each resident, based on weight, body requirements, and medical condition.

Dehydration is a serious condition resulting from inadequate fluid in the body. It can occur if residents do not drink enough liquid. It may also develop if residents put out more liquid than they take in through urination, diarrhea, vomiting, or drainage of other secretions. It can be chronic (long-term) or acute (develops sud-

BOX 8-1
Most Common Reasons for Inadequate Fluid Intake

Most residents who become dehydrated do so because of medical illness and/or:

- mental inability to ask for liquids
- physical inability to reach for or hold a cup
- inability to pour from a pitcher
- inability to drink from a straw without assistance
- physical positioning is such that the resident cannot reach water or cannot drink comfortably

Other common reasons for inadequate fluid intake

- fear of incontinence; resident deliberately withholds fluids
- resident is not thirsty; age-related changes in thirst sensation; decreased thirst response
- changes in kidneys
- trouble swallowing liquids (dysphagia)
- poor dietary intake (some foods contain as much as 80% fluid)
- lack of available fluid
- warm environmental temperature
- depression
- stomach problems
- bedrest
- immobility
- resident does not like to drink water

denly). In its acute form, dehydration can be life-threatening. The body controls the need for fluids through thirst. Unfortunately, elderly persons have a decreased sense of thirst. Thirst may not begin until dehydration has started. Elderly persons also have a decrease in total body fluid and reduced kidney function. Because of these aging changes, facility residents are at very high risk for dehydration. Like malnutrition, dehydration can and does occur in facility residents. In fact, it is the most common fluid and electrolyte problem seen in long-term care facility residents. It can be a serious condition in the elderly. Common reasons for inadequate intake of liquids are listed in Box 8-1

Identifying residents who are at risk for dehydration. Residents with the problems listed in Box 8-1 are at risk for dehydration. Other risk factors that should be monitored and reported are:

- drink less than six cups of liquid a day
- have diarrhea, vomiting, infection, or fever
- have difficulty communicating; cannot make their needs known
- are weak or tired
- take medications to remove water from the body
- do not consume the liquids on meal trays
- consume a large amount of caffeine or alcohol
- have urinary output that exceeds fluid intake
- have had recent unplanned weight loss

- have signs and symptoms of dehydration

Residents at the greatest risk of dehydration usually have one or more of the following conditions:

- female
- bedridden
- acute illness
- age 85 or older
- four or more medications
- four or more chronic illnesses

Signs and symptoms of dehydration. Dehydration may be mistaken for many other conditions in elderly adults. If it is promptly identified, it can be reversed without lasting damage. Unfortunately, it is often difficult to diagnose. Frequent or untreated dehydration can lead to permanent damage. It also contributes to other problems, such as pressure ulcers. Signs and symptoms of dehydration that you may observe include any combination of the following:

- sunken eyeballs
- dry, brown tongue
- dry mucous membranes
- furrows or lines in tongue
- dry, inelastic skin
- weight loss
- elevated temperature
- weakness, particularly in the upper body
- **lethargy** (abnormal drowsiness)
- new or worsening mental confusion
- dark, concentrated urine
- constipation
- nausea and poor appetite

(Note: This list is not all-inclusive; it includes only signs and symptoms that you may identify in your contact with residents.)

Nutrition assistant actions. Dehydration can damage the kidneys and other body systems. It is easier to prevent than treat. Pay particular attention to confused and dependent residents who cannot drink without your help. Providing extra liquids in hot weather is especially important, as extra fluids are needed to keep the body cool. Facilities identify residents who are at risk for dehydration and develop a plan of care to prevent it from developing. Become familiar with and follow each resident's hydration care plan. Nutrition assistant actions to prevent dehydration are:

- offering the resident a drink each time you make contact; set a goal, such as 2 to 4 ounces of liquid each time
- providing fluids the resident likes, at the preferred temperature (as permitted)
- drinking with the resident, if permitted
- making sure fresh water is available, that the resident can reach and comfortably drink it, and that the pitcher and cup are light enough to hold
- providing straws, if this is easier for the resident
- providing ice, if cold liquids are preferred by the resident
- providing physical assistance to pour and drink fluids, as needed
- offering ice chips, if permitted
- providing food items that contain a large amount of liquid, such as popsicles or watermelon
- alternating liquids with solids when feeding meals
- encouraging the resident to attend activities involving food and fluids
- accurately monitoring and recording intake and output, when ordered
- promptly notifying the nurse of signs and symptoms of dehydration

Measuring and Recording Fluid Intake and Output

Residents who are at high risk for dehydration and those with certain medical conditions may need special fluid balance monitoring. The facility will monitor and document how much liquid these residents take in. Output from urine, vomitus, blood, and other liquid drainage is also measured and recorded. This is called **intake and output**, or **I&O**. Taking in enough liquid each day is important for all residents, including those who are not on I&O monitoring. **Fluid intake** is *all liquid* that the resident takes into the body. This includes:

- all fluids consumed in the resident's room
- fluids consumed with meals in the dining room
- fluids taken during each medication pass
- fluids consumed during activity programs and special events
- fluids given in intravenous feedings and tube feedings (The nurse is responsible for keeping track of fluid intake given through tubes.)

When monitoring I&O, certain food items are also considered liquids and should be recorded. These are things that would become liquid if allowed to stand at room temperature, such as:

- ice cream
- sherbet
- gelatin
- pudding
- custard
- popsicles

Pureed foods and items such as applesauce and yogurt are not counted as fluid intake. Most of the liquid taken in is consumed during the day and the evening. Since there are two meals on the day shift, this is when residents consume most of the fluids.

Measuring fluid intake. The metric system is used to measure fluid intake and output. Fluid intake is measured in **milliliters** (mL) or **cubic centimeters** (cc). The two measurements are equivalent. 30 mL is equivalent to one ounce. Many long-term care facilities have historically recorded all liquids using cubic centimeters. However, in 2003, several professional organizations published lists of abbreviations that increase the risk of error because of illegible or difficult to read handwriting. The abbreviation "cc" is on this list. Because of this, facilities are in the process of changing their forms and documentation to the mL measurement. Your facility will have a chart that gives the number of milliliters in commonly used containers, such as cups, dishes, and water pitchers. You must know how to convert the commonly used measurements of ounces, pints, quarts, and gallons into metric measurements. Tables 8-1 and 8-2 list the common U.S. measurements for liquids and their metric equivalents.

When calculating how much liquid a resident drinks, you must first know how much liquid the container holds when full. You will estimate how much the resident drank, then subtract it from the total. For example, a full water glass in your facility contains 8 ounces, or 240 mL. The resident drinks half a glass, or 120 mL. 240 mL minus 120 mL equals 120 mL. You will record 120 mL under the intake column of the I&O record. Some facilities serve water in cups with accurate measurements marked on the sides.

Usually, an estimation of the amount of fluid the resident drinks is adequate. When we measure intake and output, our figures are close estimates. Sometimes the doctor will order **strict I&O**. This means that the fluid the resident consumes must be measured exactly. Using the same example above, the full water glass holds 240 mL (Figure 8-1). The resident drinks approximately half a glass. You will pour this water into a measuring device to see

TABLE 8-1
Average Container Amounts

CONTAINER	APPROXIMATE NUMBER OF OUNCES	APPROXIMATE NUMBER OF ML (CC)
Water glass	6 ounces	180 mL
Styrofoam cup	6 ounces	180 mL
Juice glass	4 ounces	120 mL
Large glass	8 ounces	240 mL
Water pitcher	32 ounces (1 quart)	1000 mL (960 mL)
Coffee or tea pot	10 ounces	300 mL
Coffee cup	5 ounces	150 mL
Milk carton	8 ounces	240 mL
Soup bowl (small)	6 ounces	180 mL
Soup bowl (large)	10 ounces	300 mL
Gelatin	4 ounces	120 mL
Ice cream cup	4 ounces	120 mL
Creamer	1 ounce	30 mL

TABLE 8-2
U.S. and Metric Equivalents

COMMON U.S. MEASUREMENT	METRIC EQUIVALENT
1 teaspoon	5 mL
1 ounce	30 mL
½ pint	250 mL
1 pint	500 mL
1 quart	1,000 mL (or 1 liter)
½ gallon	2,000 mL
1 gallon	4,000 mL

how much is left. After you do this, you find that 118 mL remains in the glass. 240 mL minus 118 mL equals 122 mL (Figure 8–1). You will record 122 mL on the I&O record. This method of measuring intake and output is more accurate, but as you can see, the figures are very close to the estimated amount in the first example. You may also measure the exact amount of fluid before and after serving the resident, if this is your facility's policy.

Each resident's intake and output is totaled and recorded at the end of every shift. The totals for all three shifts are added together and recorded once every 24 hours (Figure 8-2). You may be assigned to add the total intake at the end of your shift. Remember that most people drink 2000 to 3000 mL every 24 hours. Most facility residents should drink at least 1600 mL to 2000 mL. Drinking less than this may not be enough to meet the body's needs. If the total for your shift seems too low, inform the nurse. Your facility may have guidelines for you to follow. For example, a facility may require you to notify the nurse if the resident takes in less than 1200 mL on the day shift and 1000 mL on the second shift. Judge your estimates by the shift, knowing that most fluids are taken on the day shift.

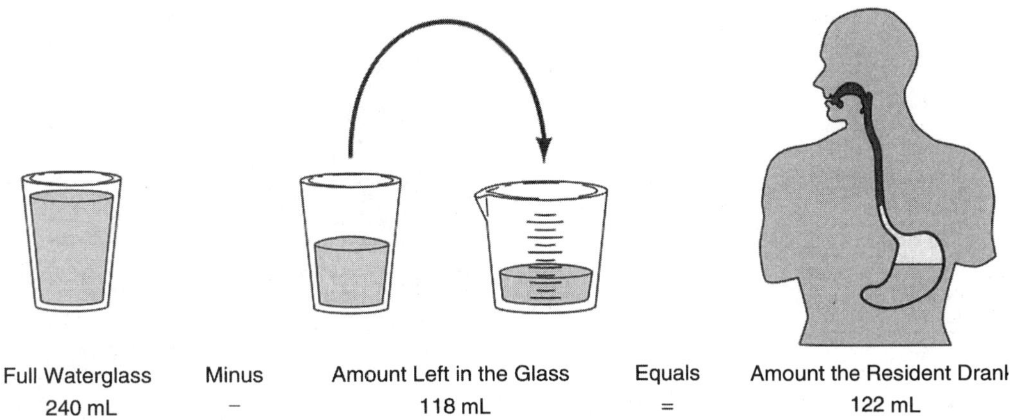

FIGURE 8-1
Liquids are carefully measured when the resident has an order for strict I&O monitoring.

Intake Section of Intake and Output Form

Time	Oral INTAKE Kind	Amount	Tube Feeding	Intravenous	Other
0700	Coffee	120 mL			
	Juice	100 mL			
	Milk	240 mL			
1000	Water	180 mL			
1200	Soup	120 mL			
	Juice	100 mL			
	Coffee	120 mL			
	Milk	240 mL			
8 Hour Total		1220 mL			
1500	Water	90 mL			
1800	Soup	200 mL			
	Milk	240 mL			
2000	Ensure	240 mL			
2210	Water	200 mL			
8 Hour Total		970 mL			
2300	Juice	120 mL			
8 Hour Total		120 mL			
24 Hour Total		2310 mL			

Worksheet
Oral Intake
1220 mL
970 mL
120 mL
Total 2310 mL

FIGURE 8-2
The oral intake is on the left side of the form. The type of fluid, time, and amount are recorded. The intake is totaled every 8 hours and cumulated every 24 hours.

Procedure 6— Measuring Fluid Intake

1. Wash your hands (or use an alcohol hand cleaner).
2. Gather supplies:
   - graduate or measuring container
   - I&O record
   - equivalent list, if equivalents not listed on I&O record
   - pen
   - scratch paper, if needed
   - calculator, if needed
3. Estimate or measure and record all fluid consumed by the resident.
4. Check all serving containers for remaining liquid.
5. Determine the amount of the serving from the equivalent list.
6. Accurately estimate (or measure) the amount of liquid remaining.
7. Subtract the amount remaining from amount of serving to determine fluid intake.
8. Record the time and amount of fluid intake on the I&O record.
9. Wash your hands (or use an alcohol hand cleaner).

Force fluids. Residents who need extra fluid often have a physician's order to **force fluids**. This does not mean that you physically force the resident to drink, but that you will encourage the resident to drink as many fluids as possible. Approaches that may be helpful for encouraging fluids include:

- Let the resident select a beverage of choice, as allowed.

- Find out what beverages the resident likes and provide them.
- Offer the resident a drink with each contact.
- Try offering fluid frequently in small amounts.
- Try offering fluid frequently in a large glass.
- Provide food items with high water content, such as popsicles and watermelon.
- If the resident is alert, have her or him set a goal for fluid intake. Help her or him achieve the goal each day.

Intake and output is usually monitored for residents who have force fluid orders. You will write down the amount the resident drinks each time.

Fluid restrictions. Sometimes residents with heart or kidney disease or other medical problems have **fluid restrictions**. Residents with fluid restrictions are allowed a very limited amount of fluid each day. The total liquid for a 24-hour period is calculated carefully. Usually, the total is divided by three shifts and the care plan lists how much fluid each shift may give the resident. The fluid given includes anything served on meal trays as well as liquids consumed on the nursing unit. Most of the nursing-unit water is used during medication passes. The day shift usually gives the largest quantity. The night shift may give only a small amount of fluid, because the resident is usually asleep. Table 8-3 gives an example of how fluid is divided.

TABLE 8-3
Allocating Fluid Intake

When establishing goals for fluid intake and fluid restrictions, intake may be divided as follows:

• day shift	½ of total 24-hour fluid goal/restriction
• second shift	⅓ of total 24-hour fluid goal/restriction
• third shift	⅙ of total 24-hour fluid goal/restriction

SERVING FRESH DRINKING WATER

You may be assigned to pass fresh drinking water to residents every 4 to 8 hours. Consult the care plan to see if the resident is allowed to have ice. In certain medical conditions, beverages are served without ice. Also check to see if residents are **NPO**. This is the medical abbreviation for "nothing by mouth." Most facilities remove the cup and water pitcher from the room while a resident is NPO. You must also learn whether the resident has special fluid orders, such as force fluids, fluid restrictions, or I&O monitoring.

The method of serving drinking water and the type of ice dispenser will vary with your facility. A few facilities serve bottled water. If residents request ice, it is delivered in a plastic sandwich bag or disposable cup. However, most facilities refill the residents' water pitchers with ice and fresh water each shift.

Guidelines for Providing Fresh Drinking Water

- Wash your hands (or use an alcohol cleanser) before beginning this procedure. If your hands become contaminated, or if you assist a resident, cleanse your hands again before continuing. Your hands remain clean if you are touching only clean items.
- Follow facility policy and good infection control practices.
- Avoid contaminating the ice scoop, ice machine, or supply of clean ice with your hands, a cup, a pitcher, or an ice scoop.

- Avoid touching the pitcher with the ice scoop when you are filling it with ice.
- Do not pour water from a cup back into a water pitcher.
- Avoid filling a pitcher or cup directly over the clean ice supply. Ice from the scoop will hit the outside of the container and fall back into the clean ice supply, causing contamination. Fill the pitcher over a plastic bag, sink, or other container.
- Offer to assist residents to take a drink of fresh water.
- Avoid mixing the pitchers and cups if there is more than one resident in the room. Pitchers and cups that are reused should be labeled with each resident's name. They are sanitized regularly in the dishwasher. Some facilities color-code the pitchers. For example, mauve is always for the bed near the window. Blue is always for the bed closest to the door. Using a color-coded system is easier than trying to return the correct pitcher to each resident after they have been washed. In any event, return the correct pitcher to each resident.
- Pick up the pitchers and send to the dietary department to be sanitized according to facility policy.

Hydration Programs

Many facilities have formal hydration programs. Some use hospitality carts twice a day to provide fluids. These programs are usually informal. Facilities may provide sugar-free beverages in the dining room or other area of the facility (Figure 8-3). Residents can help themselves to these beverages throughout the day. Sugar-free beverages are used because the area is not always monitored by staff. Some residents have diabetes and other conditions in which sugar is harmful. Some facilities make coffee available as well. However, coffee should be monitored. Unsupervised residents can spill the hot coffee, causing serious burns.

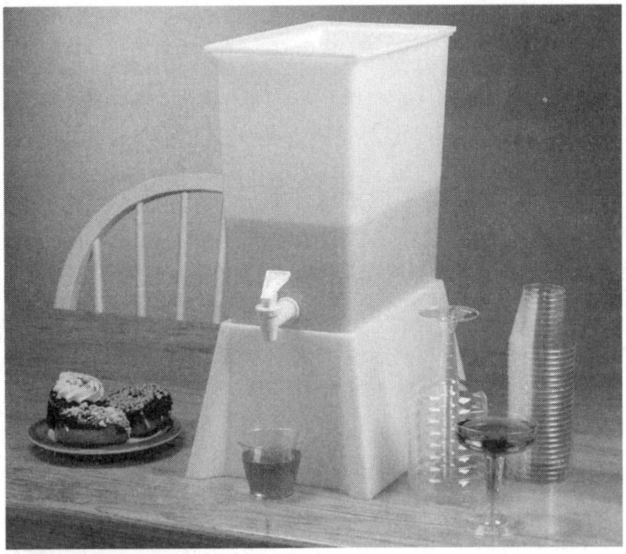

FIGURE 8-3
Residents enjoy being able to help themselves to beverages throughout the day. (Compliments of Briggs Corporation, Des Moines, IA (800) 247-2343.)

Some facilities distribute juice or other liquids several times each day. Staff members stop to offer each resident a drink. They provide assistance with drinking, if needed. All staff are responsible for providing fluids. Offer fluids as often as possible. Monitor for signs of inadequate fluid intake and dehydration, and inform the nurse. Ensuring residents receive adequate fluids is a very important responsibility!

CHAPTER REVIEW

Multiple Choice

Select the one best answer.

1. Most adults consume:
   - **a.** 100 to 500 mL of fluid daily.
   - **b.** 500 to 1000 mL of fluid daily.

c. 2000 to 3000 mL of fluid daily.
d. 4000 to 5000 mL of fluid daily.

2. Unless fluid restrictions are in place, facility residents should consume at least:
   a. 1600 to 2000 mL of fluid daily.
   b. 1000 to 1400 mL of fluid daily.
   c. 500 to 1000 mL of fluid daily.
   d. 100 to 500 mL of fluid daily.
3. The medical term for the condition that results from inadequate fluid in the body is:
   a. rehydration.
   b. dehydration.
   c. alteration of water.
   d. malnutrition.
4. Lethargy is:
   a. hyperactivity.
   b. abnormal thirst.
   c. headache.
   d. abnormal drowsiness.
5. One quart is approximately the same as:
   a. 100 mL
   b. 250 mL
   c. 500 mL
   d. 1000 mL
6. 30 mL is equivalent to:
   a. 1 teaspoon
   b. 1 ounce
   c. 1 cup
   d. 1 quart
7. 8 ounces is equivalent to:
   a. 24 mL
   b. 80 mL
   c. 240 mL
   d. 800 mL
8. 500 mL is approximately equivalent to:
   a. 1/2 pint
   b. 1 pint
   c. 1 quart
   d. 1 gallon
9. When a resident has an order to force fluids, you know this means:
   a. The nutrition assistant should force the resident to drink.
   b. The resident must consume at least one pitcher of water each shift.
   c. The nurse is responsible for administering fluids.
   d. The resident should be encouraged to drink as much as possible.
10. Residents with fluid restrictions:
    a. must drink 2000 mL to 3000 mL each day.
    b. are on I&O monitoring.
    c. should not consume more than 500 mL daily.
    d. are given fluids only by the nurse.
11. Residents who are at risk of dehydration:
    a. drink six cups of fluid each day.
    b. are always confused.
    c. have straw-colored urine.
    d. often have difficulty holding a cup.
12. Miss Phillips is on a clear liquid diet. For lunch, she drank 4 ounces of cranberry juice. She ate 100% of her 4 ounce bowl of gelatin. She drank a 6 ounce cup of tea. You will record her oral intake as:
    a. 400 mL
    b. 446 mL
    c. 680 mL
    d. 820 mL
13. You filled Mrs. King's water pitcher at 8:00 A.M. The pitcher contained 1000 mL of water and ice. At 2:30 P.M., when you collect the intake and output, there is 335 mL remaining in the pitcher. You will record Mrs. King's water intake for your shift as:
    a. 856 mL
    b. 765 mL
    c. 665 mL
    d. 586 mL

UNIT 9

Observation and Reporting

OBJECTIVES

- Spell and define key terms.
- List at least 12 observations to report to the nurse regarding residents' nutrition and hydration.
- Define objective reporting and state why this is important.

OBSERVING RESIDENTS

You are responsible for making observations about residents and reporting them to the nurse. This is an important responsibility. You are in an excellent position to notice changes because of your close working relationship with residents. Residents have unique conditions and behaviors. They do not change much from one day to the next. As you work with residents, you will learn many "normals," such as their skin condition and temperature, mental status, and self-feeding ability. Sudden changes may indicate an emergency. Gradual changes may indicate the onset of illness or infection. Report any changes from the resident's normal condition.

You will use your senses to make observations. Many changes are things that you can see. You may notice changes in movement, position, facial expression, or color. They suggest pain or another problem. You will hear some changes, such as noisy breathing and things residents tell you. Your sense of smell is useful to detect unusual odors that suggest a problem. You will note temperature changes or moisture on the skin with your sense of touch. Observing the resident is a continuous process. If you see, feel, hear, or smell anything that seems abnormal, inform the nurse. Changes that seem insignificant may indicate a problem. Your responsibility is to report them to the nurse, who will assess the resident and select the course of action. Overall, you should report:

- changes in the resident's mood, behavior, or mental status
- comments or complaints the resident makes about his or her condition, such as pain, dizziness, numbness, and so forth
- changes in the resident's breathing
- changes in the resident's skin color
- lips, fingernail beds, mucous membranes in mouth blue or blue-gray in appearance
- resident complaints
- changes in the resident's body that you can see
- what you observe using your senses of hearing, touch, smell, and sight

- care that works well for the resident
- approaches that are not working for the resident

If you report observations to the nurse and the resident's condition seems to worsen, inform the nurse again. Box 9-1 provides an overview of changes to report for nutrition and hydration. Box 9-2 lists special observations to report for residents with diabetes. Box 9-3 details changes in mental status that are important to report.

BOX 9-1
Observations to Make and Report Related to Resident Nutrition

Sores, ulcers, or white patches inside the mouth
Difficulty chewing or swallowing food
Complaints of pain, constipation, diarrhea, bleeding
Frequent belching
Changes in appetite
Excessive thirst
Unusual smell to breath
Complaints of indigestion
Excessive gas (flatus)
Nausea, vomiting
Choking
Abdominal pain
Abdominal distention (swelling)
Oral bleeding
Abnormal appearance of teeth or gums, obvious dental pain
Dentures that slip when the resident eats
Broken teeth or dentures

Increase or decrease in food intake
Residents who do not adhere to restricted diet or fluid restriction
Improvement or decline of self-care ability
Refusal to accept meals, supplements, snacks, liquids
Refusal to accept food substitute for meat or vegetable
Meal intake of less than 50% (or 75%, according to facility policy)

Observations to make and report related to resident hydration
Drinking less than 6 cups of liquid a day
Dry mouth, lips, tongue, mucous membranes
Cracked lips
Sunken eyes
New onset of difficulty swallowing liquids
Coughing, choking, gagging when swallowing liquids
Skin hot to touch, suggesting fever
New onset of mental confusion or worsening mental confusion
Weak or tired
Lethargy, difficulty staying awake

Additional signs and symptoms of dehydration and fluid balance problems listed in Unit 8

BOX 9-2
Important Observations of Diabetic Residents

Inadequate food intake
Eating food not allowed on diet
Refusal of meals, supplements, or snacks
Nausea, vomiting, or diarrhea
Inadequate fluid intake
Excessive activity
Complaints of dizziness, shakiness, racing heart

Signs and Symptoms of Abnormally High Blood Sugar (Hyperglycemia, Diabetic Coma)	Signs and Symptoms of Abnormally Low Blood Sugar (Hypoglycemia, Insulin Shock)
Nausea, vomiting	Complaints of hunger, weakness, dizziness, shakiness
Weakness	Feeling faint or lightheaded
Headache	Skin cold, moist, clammy, pale
Fruity smell to breath	Rapid, shallow respirations
Hot, dry, flushed skin	Nervousness and excitement
Labored respirations	Unconsciousness
Drowsiness	
Mental confusion	
Unconsciousness	

BOX 9-3
Mental Status Observations to Make and Report

Changes in consciousness, awareness, or alertness
Changes in mood, behavior, or emotional status
Changes in orientation to person, place, time, season
Changes in communication
Changes in memory
Excessive drowsiness
Changes in ability to respond verbally or nonverbally
Sleepiness for no apparent reason
Sudden onset of mental confusion
Threats of suicide or harm to self or others

PAIN

Pain is not normal. If residents complain of pain, inform the nurse. Body language may be the first clue that a resident is having pain (Figure 9-1). Look for pain on movement, facial expressions, crying, moaning, and unusual positioning. The resident may withdraw when touched. The resident may favor one extremity. She or he may become irritable, fatigued, or withdrawn. The resident may refuse to eat. Often, the resident acts opposite of normal. For example, a resident who is normally

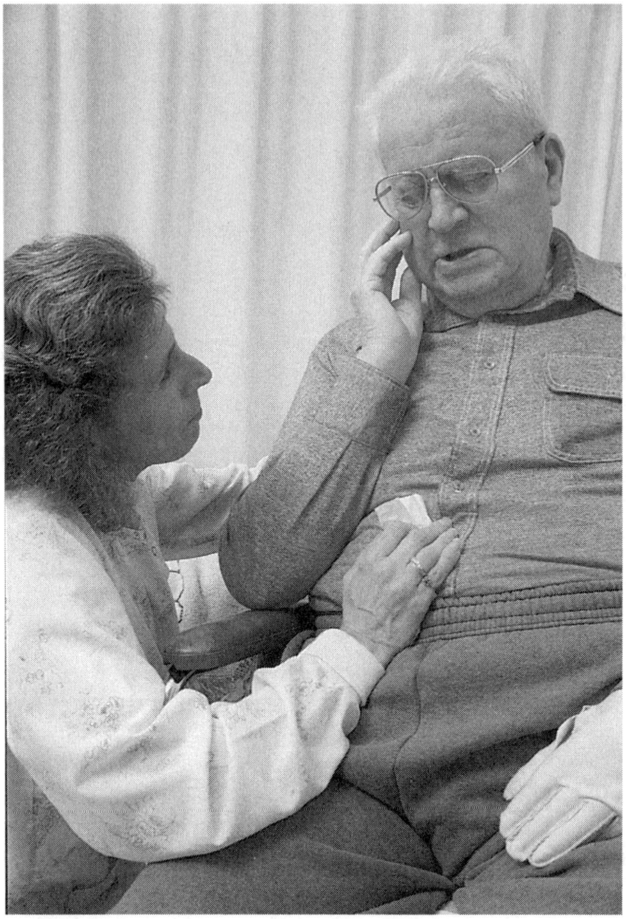

FIGURE 9-1
This resident's body language suggests he is having severe pain. Unrelieved pain contributes to complications of immobility, decreases quality of life, and may cause hopelessness, anxiety, depression, and a feeling of helplessness. Pain may cause acting out, crying, and other strange, belligerent, or combative behavior. It is a major preventable public health problem that slows recovery in individuals with acute illness, complicates chronic illness, and increases health care costs. Relieving pain is an important nursing responsibility. Report body language and other signs of pain to the nurse promptly.

very quiet becomes noisy. The agitated and combative resident becomes quiet and nonverbal. A friendly and outgoing resident cries easily and withdraws. Always suspect pain if the resident's behavior changes. Report your observations to the nurse compared with the normal behavior for the resident.

Although many residents with pain display outward signs through their body language and behavior, avoid making assumptions about the presence or absence of pain if the resident is laughing, talking, or sleeping. For example, you may assume that residents who are smiling or laughing cannot be in pain, believing that they should be grimacing, frowning, or crying. This is untrue. Some residents may appear comfortable while having severe pain. The resident's self-report of pain is the most accurate and reliable indicator of pain, and should be believed. Some residents may use different terms to identify pain, such as "sore," "hurt," and "tender." Notify the nurse if a resident complains of pain.

TYPES OF OBSERVATIONS

Objective observations are factual. They can be observed by others. They are made by seeing, hearing, feeling, touching, and smelling. **Subjective** observations may or may not be factual. Subjective observations are based on what you think or information the resident gives you that may or may not be true. Reporting that the resident did not eat lunch is an objective observation. Reporting that the resident ate a good breakfast and probably was not hungry at lunchtime is subjective. It reflects what you think. In fact, the resident may have felt nauseated, had pain, been upset, or had another reason for not eating. Avoid making assumptions. Report factual information to the nurse. If in doubt about reporting something, err on the side of safety. Inform the nurse.

Reporting Observations

Information reported to the nurse must be objective. Report observations and changes in condition promptly. You are responsible for reporting the information. The nurse is responsible for interpreting it, based on his or her assessment of the resident. If the resident changes further after you have reported to the nurse, report again. Do not assume that he or she knows there is a problem. The nurse may have forgotten to check the resident. The resident's condition may have changed.

You will also report to the nurse when you leave the unit for any reason and when you return. You will report off at the end of your shift. Likewise, you can expect to receive a report when you receive your assignment at the beginning of your shift, and periodically if residents' conditions change.

CHAPTER REVIEW

Multiple Choice

Select the one best answer.

1. An objective observation is one that you:
   a. think or feel.
   b. can weigh.
   c. can observe.
   d. measure.
2. A subjective observation is one that you:
   a. measure.
   b. can weigh.
   c. can see.
   d. think or feel.
3. Which of the following would you report to the nurse?
   a. Mr. Hargett is always a picky eater. He often eats 50%. Today he refuses all food and fluids.
   b. Mrs. Lampe is on a regular diet. Today she requested a second piece of cake.
   c. Miss Espinosa said she did not like beets and requested the vegetable substitute.
   d. Mr. Bugee normally eats 100% of his meal. He ate 96% of his lunch.
4. Mrs. Dullea is a pleasantly confused resident who normally drinks all her fluids. She likes sugar-free punch and often asks for seconds. The resident is on I&O. Today, she drank 75 mL at breakfast and 30 mL at lunch. She did not drink the sugar-free punch at lunch. It is time for you to leave. You should:
   a. Remind the resident to drink more at supper.
   b. Document the resident's intake and notify the nurse verbally.
   c. Document the resident's fluid intake, punch out, and go home.
   d. Ask a nursing assistant to push fluids on Mrs. Dullea this afternoon.
5. You just attended an inservice on resident rights. The social worker said residents had the right to refuse to follow their therapeutic diets. Mr. Calzaretta is an alert resident on a diabetic diet. You know he gets an insulin shot every day. Another resident did not eat her cake, so Mr. Calzaretta ate it. Later, you saw him at the vending machines buying a candy bar and a regular soft drink. You know the resident has the right to eat and drink whatever he wants. You should:
   a. Do nothing, since the resident has the right to eat and drink whatever he wants.
   b. Take the candy and soda away and tell the resident he should buy sugar-free items instead.
   c. Say nothing about this to anyone because of the resident's right to privacy.
   d. Inform the nurse of the resident's food and drink intake.
6. Mrs. Khoo is on a low-cholesterol diet. She ate 100% of breakfast and 80% of her lunch. She said she was full and refused the substitutes. It is

almost time for you to leave for the day. You should:

a. Document the resident's intake and go home.

b. Offer the resident a snack before leaving for the day.

c. Tell her nursing assistant to give the resident extra food.

d. Inform the nurse that the resident did not eat well.

7. Mr. Traa is an underweight resident on a low-sodium diet. He ate 70% at breakfast. At lunch, he says he is "starved." He asks for seconds of the green beans, dinner roll, and fruited gelatin. You should:

a. Tell him he cannot have seconds because of the low-sodium diet.

b. Give him what he asks for, as these things are permitted on his diet.

c. Tell the resident to wait a few minutes and see if he feels full.

d. Ask the resident's nursing assistant what to do.

8. Mrs. Nikkinen grimaces when she drinks a cold beverage. She tells you it hit the wrong spot, and her tooth is "a little tender," but that she will be all right. She denies pain. You should:

a. Do nothing, as the resident tells you she is fine.

b. Ask a nursing assistant to check the resident right away.

c. Inform the nurse of the resident's reaction and comments.

d. Exchange the cold beverage for a warm beverage.

9. Miss Ronzani is a pleasantly confused resident who is quiet and cooperative. She tells female residents and staff how pretty they are. She is usually disoriented to time and place. However, she is so sweet and friendly that everyone likes her. When you try to feed her breakfast, she is very agitated and upset. She will not eat her food. She warns you there are spiders crawling all over the walls, and rats running around on the tables. She fears they will come and bite her and take her food. What action will you take?

a. Reassure the resident that you will protect her and encourage her to eat.

b. Tell the resident you have killed the rats and spiders and they are gone now.

c. Tell the resident she is imagining things and that she must eat her meal.

d. Reassure the resident and inform the nurse of a change in mental status.

10. Mr. Calzaretta is not feeling well. He received his insulin shot, but says he does not want to eat. The nurse tells you to keep your eyes on him. Signs and symptoms of low blood sugar to watch for include:

a. fruity smell to breath.

b. feeling nervous and dizzy.

c. hot, dry, flushed skin.

d. headache and nausea.

APPENDIX A

DOCUMENTING PERCENTAGE OF MEALS CONSUMED

Many methods are used for documenting percentage of meals consumed. Wait until each resident has finished eating before calculating meal intake. Documenting appetite is more than eyeballing the food tray and estimating how much of the food was eaten. Instead, you must document the percentage of the significant food items on the tray. Your facility will select a method for calculating resident meal intake. Every staff member and volunteer should use the same method of calculation and documentation. The system should also be used for snacks, nourishments, and supplements. Some facilities record percentages of each individual food item on the tray for residents with weight loss, or when accurate intake recording is essential. Some facilities have a policy such as the one below to promptly identify and act on inadequate meal intake.

- If a resident consumes 50% or less in any three meals over a three-day period of time, his or her name is added to a special "watch" list. Residents whose names are listed will be closely observed and assisted (as needed) over the next three days to identify the problem. The dietary manager and registered dietitian will assess the resident and make recommendations to improve intake.
- Look at each item on the tray and estimate how much the resident has eaten.
- Add the points and document as the percentage consumed.

The following are examples of different systems for evaluating food intake.

Point Method One

The point method of calculating meal intake assigns a point value to each item on the tray. Staff will:

- Add the number of points the resident has eaten.
- Record the number of points as a percentage on the food acceptance record.
- Use the following to calculate food intake:

Point Method One

• Coffee, tea, water, condiments = 0 points
Breakfast
Toast = 20
Juice = 20
Milk = 20
Eggs = 20
Cereal = 20
Total = 100
Lunch and Dinner
Bread = 10
Meat/Entree = 50
Vegetable or Soup = 20
Dessert = 20
Total = 100
Good = 75–100 points
Fair = 50–74 points
Poor = 0–49 points

Point Method Two

- Coffee, water, tea, and condiments equal no points.
- Each food item served equals one point.
- If the resident consumes all food items in the amount served, the resident consumes 100% of the meal.
  Example:
  - breakfast consists of four items: eggs, toast with butter, milk, juice, coffee.
  - eggs = 1, toast with butter = 1, milk = 1, juice = 1, coffee = 0
- If the resident consumes two of four food items served, then 50% of the meal is consumed.
  Example:
  - resident eats all toast, drinks all milk. Leaves the other items = 50%
- If partial amount of an item is consumed, use the following for giving points:
  - three-fourths of a food item is consumed, give one point
  - for one-half consumed, give 0.5 point
  - for one-fourth or less, give no points
- Total the points consumed. Multiply × 100
- Divide by the number of items served for that meal (such as four in breakfast above) to give the percentage of meal consumed. Example for dinner: coffee (no points), milk, rice, chicken, roll and butter, and dessert. Meal equals a possible 5 points. The resident drinks none of the milk, eats half of the rice, the entire chicken breast, all of the dessert and none of the bread. Point total consumed: $2.5 \times 100 = 250 \div 5 = 50\%$
- Record the percentage on the food acceptance record.

Percent Method One

When the meal is complete, visually evaluate the resident's total food intake:

- Estimate the percent of food eaten based on the amount of food remaining
- Coffee, tea, water, condiments = 0 points
- Record in increments of 0–25–50–75–100%
- Document the percentage on the food acceptance record

Percent Method Two

When the meal is complete, visually evaluate the resident's total food intake:

- Estimate the percent of each food item eaten based on the amount of food remaining, using the chart on page 107
- Coffee, tea, water, condiments = 0 points
- Add all food items eaten
- Document the total as the percentage on the food acceptance record

Percent Method Three

When the meal is complete, visually evaluate the resident's total food intake:

- Using the chart on page 107, estimate the percent of food eaten based on the amount of food remaining
- Coffee, tea, water, condiments = 0 points
- Document the percentage on the food acceptance record

CALORIE COUNTS AND FOOD INTAKE STUDIES

The physician or dietitian may order special food intake studies for residents who

Percent Method Two

	FOOD ITEM	PERCENTAGE OF MEAL
Breakfast		
	eggs	35%
	eggs and bacon	40%
	eggs and sausage	45%
	toast *or* cereal	30%
	milk	20%
	fruit juice	15%
Dinner and Supper	meat group, including eggs, main dish, legumes	50%
	fruit group, including dessert items	15%
	bread or cereal group	10%
	vegetable group	15%
	fluids	10%

Percent Method Three

Breakfast	
Egg, cheese, or cottage cheese	50%
Hot or cold cereal	30%
Bread	10%
Bacon, ham, or sausage	10%
Total	100%

Occasionally, a resident will request no protein foods (eggs, meat, cheese, cottage cheese) at breakfast. Please reassign the percentages to the other items on the tray and document accordingly.

Lunch and Supper	
Meat, egg, cheese, or cottage cheese	40%
Starchy vegetable	20%
Vegetable or salad	20%
Bread	10%
Dessert	10%
Total	100%

The meat and starchy vegetables may be combined in some dishes, such as casseroles. If so, add the point value for these items together to total 60%. Sandwiches are also 60% because the two breads are the starchy vegetable. An additional bread item such as crackers may also be served at the meal.

are at risk of malnutrition or who have special nutritional needs. The resident's food intake is carefully recorded for a period of time, usually three days. The food intake is analyzed for nutritional adequacy and number of calories consumed. The dietitian uses this information to plan a diet to meet the resident's special medical needs.

If the physician orders a food intake study, a special food documentation form (Figure A1) is prepared and placed in a designated location. The study usually begins with the breakfast meal on the day after the physician writes the order. In some facilities, each food item is weighed or measured. At the end of each meal, you will accurately record the resident's food intake on the form. Facility policies vary on how food intake is documented, but this is usually done by recording an accurate percentage of each individual meal item. You will also accurately document intake of all snacks, liquid nutritional beverages, and food items brought in by visitors.

At the end of the study period, the form is returned to the dietitian. He or she will

Diet ____________________

CALORIE/PROTEIN SUMMARY

RESIDENT ____ ROOM # ____________________

DAY 1					DAY 2					DAY 3				
DATE ___/___/___					DATE ___/___/___					DATE ___/___/___				
	% 0–25	% 25–50	% 50–75	% 75–100		% 0–25	% 25–50	% 50–75	% 75–100		% 0–25	% 25–50	% 50–75	% 75–100
Breakfast					**Breakfast**					**Breakfast**				
Meat					Meat					Meat				
Milk					Milk					Milk				
Fruit					Fruit					Fruit				
Starch					Starch					Starch				
Fat					Fat					Fat				
Other					Other					Other				
AM Supp.					AM Supp.					AM Supp.				
Noon Meal					**Noon Meal**					**Noon Meal**				
Meat					Meat					Meat				
Milk					Milk					Milk				
Juice					Juice					Juice				
Starch					Starch					Starch				
Vegetable					Vegetable					Vegetable				
Bread					Bread					Bread				
Fat					Fat					Fat				
Dessert					Dessert					Dessert				
Other					Other					Other				
PM Supp.					PM Supp.					PM Supp.				
Evening Meal					**Evening Meal**					**Evening Meal**				
Meat					Meat					Meat				
Milk					Milk					Milk				
Juice					Juice					Juice				
Starch					Starch					Starch				
Vegetable					Vegetable					Vegetable				
Bread					Bread					Bread				
Fat					Fat					Fat				
Dessert					Dessert					Dessert				
Other					Other					Other				
PM Supp.					PM Supp.					PM Supp.				
Total Kcal					**Total Kcal**					**Total Kcal**				
Total Pro					**Total Pro**					**Total Pro**				
Avg. for 3 days Kcal:							**Avg. Protein for 3 days:**							

PLEASE RETURN COMPLETED FORM TO NUTRITION CARE MANAGER

FIGURE APPENDIX A-1
The calorie count provides an accurate picture of the resident's calorie and nutrient intake over a three-day period. The information is used to adjust the resident's diet and nutritional plan of care.

use the information to calculate the amount of protein, carbohydrates, fat, and calories the resident consumed each day. In some facilities, nutrient, vitamin, and mineral intake is also calculated. The dietitian will use this information to make recommendations for adjusting the resident's diet and nutritional plan of care. The results of the study and dietitian's recommendations are communicated to the physician, who may change the diet order. He or she may also order extra vitamin or mineral supplements needed by the resident. Completing a food intake or calorie count study requires a team effort, good communication, and accurate documentation.

ESTIMATING FLUID INTAKE

When calculating I&O, you must consider how much fluid is in the container. For example, an 8 ounce glass does not contain 8 ounces of fluid unless it is filled all the way to the top. Filling containers to the top is not practical in the long-term care facility because it increases the risk of spilling. The chart on page 111 is based on actual container size. The chart on page 112 provides estimates of fluid when the containers are reasonably full, but not completely ful.

Procedure 7—Serving Fresh Drinking Water in Clean Pitchers

1. Obtain a list of residents with special fluid orders and preferences, such as nothing by mouth (NPO) or no ice.
   - Obtain a clean utility cart.
2. Push cart down hallway. Stop at each room.
   - Knock on each door and wait for a response.
   - Identify yourself, greet the resident, identify each resident, and explain what you are doing.
3. Collect each pitcher and cup. Empty at the sink.
   - Record fluid intake on I&O record as appropriate.
4. Take pitchers and glasses to the kitchen for washing.
5. Wash your hands (or use an alcohol hand cleaner).
6. Collect clean pitchers and cups from the kitchen.
7. Gather supplies on clean utility cart.
   - Clean pitchers with lids, cups
   - Container of clean ice
   - Clean ice scoop in plastic bag or covered container
   - Large plastic trash bag attached to side of cart and hanging open to catch falling ice
   - Pitcher of clean water (or fill pitchers at sink, according to facility policy)
   - Extra cups and straws
8. Fill clean pitchers with ice and water, according to facility policy. Avoid contaminating ice machine, ice scoop, or ice.
9. Push cart down hallway. Stop at each room.
   - Knock on each door and wait for a response.
   - Identify yourself, greet the resident, identify each resident and explain what you are doing.
   - Leave a clean pitcher of fresh water and a clean glass at each resident's bedside. Make sure you return pitcher to the correct resident.
   - Check and follow the list of special fluid orders and residents' preferences for ice, straws.
10. Offer and pour a glass of water for each resident and encourage fluid intake. Assist, if needed. If you assist a resident, wash your hands

Reference Table for Fluid Intake

	PERCENT CONSUMED				
BEVERAGE	**0%**	**25%**	**50%**	**75%**	**100%**
Juice/Water 4 oz	0 mL	30 mL	60 mL	90 mL	120 mL
Juice/Water 6 oz	0 mL	45 mL	90 mL	135 mL	180 mL
Juice/Water 8 oz	0 mL	60 mL	120 mL	180 mL	240 mL
Juice/Water 10 oz	0 mL	70 mL	140 mL	210 mL	300mL
Juice/Water 12 oz	0 mL	90 mL	180 mL	270 mL	360 mL
Milk 8 oz	0 mL	60 mL	120 mL	180 mL	240 mL
Mighty Shake 6 oz	0 mL	45 mL	90 mL	135 mL	180 mL
Shake Up 8 oz	0 mL	60 mL	120 mL	180 mL	240 mL
Supplement 6 oz	0 mL	45 mL	90 mL	135 mL	180 mL
Supplement 8 oz	0 mL	60 mL	120 mL	180 mL	240 mL
Soda 8 oz	0 mL	60 mL	120 mL	180 mL	240 mL
Soda 12 oz	0 mL	90 mL	180 mL	270 mL	360 mL
Soda 16 oz	0 mL	120 mL	240 mL	360 mL	480 mL
Ice Cream 4 oz	0 mL	30 mL	60 mL	90 mL	120 mL
Coffee 8 oz	0 mL	60 mL	120 mL	180 mL	240 mL
Soup Cup 6 oz	0 mL	45 mL	90 mL	135 mL	180 mL
Soup Bowl 10 oz	0 mL	70 mL	140 mL	210 mL	300 mL
Estimate serving sizes based on size, type, and fill of container.					

Metric Volume of Containers

METRIC VOLUME	**EXACT METRIC VOLUME**
1 liter (l or L) = 1000 milliliters (cc)	½ pint = 236 mL (250 mL)
1 milliliter = 1000 microliters	1 pint (pt) = 473 mL (500 mL)
1 teaspoon (tsp) = 5 mL	
1 tablespoon (T or tbs) = 15 mL	
2 tablespoons = 30 mL	
1 measuring cup = 240 mL	

(or use an alcohol hand cleaner) before continuing.

11. Record fluid intake on I&O record, if ordered.
12. Upon completion of procedure, wash your hands (or use an alcohol hand cleaner). Return the cart and supplies to the proper storage area.

GUIDELINES FOR HAND HYGIENE

In 2002, the Centers for Disease Control and Prevention (CDC) published the results of extensive handwashing studies, as well as new recommendations for cleansing hands. Each recommendation is catego-

Estimating Fluid Intake

OUNCES/ CONTAINER SIZE	MILLILITERS IN CONTAINER, SUCH AS MILK CARTON, SODA POP, ICE CREAM CARTON	ESTIMATED MILLILITERS IN FILLED CONTAINER, SUCH AS GLASS OF MILK, CUP OF COFFEE, BOWL OF SOUP
½ fl. ounce	15 mL	
1 fl. ounce	30 mL	
1½ fl. ounce	45 mL	
2 fl. ounce	60 mL	
3 fl. ounce	90 mL	75 mL
4 fl. ounce	120 mL	105 mL
5 fl. ounce	150 mL	135 mL
6 fl. ounce	180 mL	165 mL
7 fl. ounce	210 mL	195 mL
8 fl. ounce	240 mL	225 mL
9 fl. ounce	270 mL	255 mL
10 fl. ounce	300 mL	285 mL
11 fl. ounce	330 mL	315 mL
12 fl. ounce	360 mL	345 mL
13 fl. ounce	390 mL	375 mL
14 fl. ounce	420 mL	405 mL
15 fl. ounce	450 mL	435 mL
16 fl. ounce	480 mL	465 mL
17 fl. ounce	510 mL	495 mL
18 fl. ounce	540 mL	525 mL
19 fl. ounce	570 mL	555 mL
20 fl. ounce	600 mL	585 mL
Remember to adjust your calculations to the amount in the container. For example, a 4 ounce juice glass may actually contain only 3 to 3½ ounces of juice, since it is not filled to the top of the glass.		

rized on the basis of existing scientific data, rationale, applicability, and economic impact. The CDC system for categorizing recommendations is:

Category IA. Strongly recommended for implementation and strongly supported by well-designed experimental, clinical, or epidemiologic studies.

Category IB. Strongly recommended

Category IC. Required for implementation, as mandated by federal or state regulation or standard.

Category II. Suggested for implementation

No recommendation. Unresolved issue.

Recommendations

1. Indications for handwashing and cleansing

Special Dietary Requirements of Cultural and Religious Groups in the United States

RELIGION/GROUP	FOOD REQUIREMENTS AND PROHIBITIONS
Adventist, Seventh Day	Alcohol, coffee, and tea are prohibited. A vegetarian diet is encouraged.
American Indian	In some tribes, sharing food is customary. Explain to visitors that they should not share the resident's food in the health care facility. After prayer and certain ceremonies, berries, corn, and dried meat are consumed. These foods may be provided by family members or other members of the tribe.
Buddhist	Buddhists do not eat meat.
Catholic	Some residents do not eat meat on Fridays and other holy days. Most do not eat meat on Fridays during Lent. Avoid food for one hour before Communion.
Chinese American	Believe in the balance of heat and cold in the body and use food to maintain this balance, as well as treating disease. Rice and noodles are staples in the diet. Eat very little meat. Meat is usually mixed with cooked vegetables. Family members may bring in special foods to treat certain illnesses. Also use herbs and herb preparations to treat illnesses.
Christian Scientist	Alcohol prohibited. Some abstain from coffee and tea.
Church of Jesus Christ of Latter Day Saints (LDS or Mormon)	Alcohol, coffee, tea, beverages with caffeine not allowed.
Hindu	Many Hindus are vegetarians. Most do not eat beef. A light meal is eaten for breakfast, a heavy meal for lunch, and a light meal for supper. Dietary customs state the right hand is used for eating and the left hand for toileting and personal hygiene.
Islam (Muslim)	Pork, pork products, and carnivorous animals are not allowed. Other meat products must be slaughtered in a certain way. Some do not eat seafood without fins or scales. Most avoid products with lard, gelatin, rennet, whey, and vanilla extract (which may contain alcohol). They have various fast days, but those who are sick are not required to fast. The right hand is used for eating. Alcohol is not allowed.
Jewish	Predatory fowl, shellfish, and pork are not allowed. Fish with fins and scales are permitted. Other types of fish not allowed. Some Jewish residents request kosher food, which requires very special preparation. Milk and meat are not eaten together. Special requirements for dishes and flatware during some religious holidays.
Mexican American	Prefer fresh natural ingredients in food preparation. Beans, corn tortillas, and rice are staples of the diet. Tomatoes are used extensively in preparation of sauces. Food is highly spiced with onions, cilantro, and chilies. Many prefer tortillas with meals instead of bread. Mexican Americans believe that the properties of some diseases are hot or cold. Foods are served to complement the hot or cold disease state. The terms do not refer to food temperature, but rather to the effect the food has on the body.
Puerto Ricans	Some observe traditional coffee time at 10:00 A.M. and 3:00 P.M. Coffee is traditionally prepared with boiled milk and sugar. Rice, beans, and plantains are served with most meals. Do not eat red meat or chicken during certain religious events.

- When hands are visibly dirty or contaminated or are visibly soiled with blood or other body fluids, wash hands with either a regular soap and water or an antimicrobial soap and water (IA).
- If hands are not visibly soiled, use an alcohol-based hand rub for routinely cleansing hands in all other clinical situations (IA).
- Alternatively, wash hands with an antimicrobial soap and water in all clinical situations (IB).
- Cleanse hands before having direct contact with patients (IB).
- Cleanse hands after contact with a patient's intact skin (e.g., when taking a pulse or blood pressure, and lifting a patient) (IB).
- Cleanse hands after contact with body fluids or excretions, mucous membranes, nonintact skin, and wound dressings if hands are not visibly soiled (IA).
- Cleanse hands if moving from a contaminated-body site to a clean-body site during patient care (II).
- Cleanse hands after contact with inanimate objects (including medical equipment) in the immediate vicinity of the patient (II).
- Cleanse hands after removing gloves (IB).
- Before eating and after using a restroom, wash hands with a regular soap and water or with an antimicrobial soap and water (IB). *(Note: In this situation regular handwashing is the recommended technique instead of using an alcohol preparation.)*
- Antimicrobial-impregnated wipes (i.e., towelettes) may be considered as an alternative to washing hands with regular soap and water. Because they are not as effective as alcohol-based hand rubs or washing hands with an antimicrobial soap and water for reducing bacterial counts on the hands of workers, they are not a substitute for using an alcohol-based hand rub or antimicrobial soap (IB).
- No recommendation can be made regarding the routine use of nonalcohol-based hand rubs for hand hygiene in health-care settings. Unresolved issue.

2. Hand-hygiene technique
   - When cleansing hands with an alcohol-based hand rub, apply product to palm of one hand and rub hands together, covering all surfaces of hands and fingers, until hands are dry (IB).
   - Follow the manufacturer's recommendations regarding the volume of product to use.
   - When washing hands with soap and water, wet hands first with water, apply an amount of product recommended by the manufacturer to hands, and rub hands together vigorously for at least 15 seconds, covering all surfaces of the hands and fingers. Rinse hands with water and dry thoroughly with a disposable towel. Use towel to turn off the faucet (IB).
   - Avoid using hot water, because repeated exposure to hot water may increase the risk of skin irritation (IB).
   - Liquid, bar, leaflet, or powdered forms of plain soap are acceptable when washing hands with a regular soap and water. When bar soap is used, soap racks that facilitate drainage and small bars of soap should be used (II).
   - Multiple-use cloth towels of the hanging or roll type are not recommended for use in health-care settings (II).

3. Other Recommendations
   - Do not add soap to a partially empty soap dispenser. This practice of "topping off" dispensers can lead to bacterial contamination of soap (IA).
   - Workers should use hand lotions or creams to reduce the risk of irritation associated with hand antisepsis or handwashing (IA).
   - Do not wear artificial fingernails or extenders when having direct contact with patients at high risk (IA).
   - Keep natural nails tips less than ¼-inch long (II)
   - Wear gloves when contact with blood or other potentially infectious materials, mucous membranes, and nonintact skin could occur (IC).
   - Remove gloves after caring for a patient. Do not wear the same pair of gloves for the care of more than one patient, and do not wash gloves between uses with different patients (IB).
   - Encourage patients and their families to remind workers to cleanse their hands (II).
   - Store supplies of alcohol-based hand rubs in cabinets or areas approved for flammable materials (IC).

Source: Excerpted from: CDC Guideline for Hand Hygiene in Health Care Settings, *Morbidity and Mortality Weekly Report* October 25, 2002 / Vol. 51 / No. RR-16.

APPENDIX B

Skills Checklist for Procedures 1–7

PERFORMANCE REVIEW CHECKLIST

Procedure 1
Procedure: Handwashing
Name of Nutrition Assistant ______________________
Date(s) of Program ______________ to ______________ Total number of hours satisfactorily completed _________
Social Security # or Other Identifying Information of Nutrition Assistant ______________________________
Program Code Number (if any) ___________ S = Satisfactory Performance U = Unsatisfactory Performance
Place a full signature to correspond with each set of initials appearing below:

INITIALS	CORRESPONDING SIGNATURE OF INSTRUCTOR	TITLE

PROCEDURE GUIDELINES	S/U	DATE	INITIALS	S/U	DATE	INITIALS
1. Turns on warm water using paper towel.						
2. Wets hands. Keeps fingertips pointed down.						
3. Applies soap from the dispenser.						
4. Rubs hands together vigorously to create a lather.						
• Rubs hands together in a circular motion for 15 seconds.						
• Rubs all surfaces of the hands. Washes well between fingers.						
• Keeps fingertips pointed down.						
• Does not touch inside of sink or faucet handles.						
5. Rubs fingernails against the palm of the opposite hand. Cleans nails with brush or orange stick if they are soiled.						
6. Rinses hands from wrists to the fingertips. Keeps the fingers pointed down.						
7. Dries hands with a paper towel.						
8. Uses clean, dry paper towel to turn off the faucet.						
Does not touch faucet handles with hands.						
9. Discards paper towel properly.						

Passed Skill _________ Failed Skill _________

______________________________________ ______________
Instructor Signature Date

______________________________________ ______________
Student Signature Date

PERFORMANCE REVIEW CHECKLIST

Procedure 2
Procedure: Applying and Removing Gloves
Name of Nutrition Assistant ____________________
Date(s) of Program ____________ to ____________ Total number of hours satisfactorily completed ________
Social Security # or Other Identifying Information of Nutrition Assistant ____________________
Program Code Number (if any) __________ S = Satisfactory Performance U = Unsatisfactory Performance
Place a full signature to correspond with each set of initials appearing below:

INITIALS	CORRESPONDING SIGNATURE OF INSTRUCTOR	TITLE

PROCEDURE GUIDELINES	S/U	DATE	INITIALS	S/U	DATE	INITIALS
Applying Disposable Gloves						
1. Washes hands (or uses alcohol hand cleaner).						
2. Removes clean gloves from the box.						
3. Puts hands into the gloves, adjusts the fingers for comfort and fit.						
4. Pulls the cuff of gloves up and adjusts them over wrists.						
Removing Disposable Gloves						
1. Grasps outside of glove on nondominant hand at cuff. Pulls glove off so the inside of glove faces outward. Avoids touching wrist with fingers of glove.						
2. Places glove into palm of hand that is still gloved.						
3. Puts fingers on ungloved hand *inside* cuff of gloved hand. Pulls glove off inside out. The first glove removed should be inside second glove.						
4. Discards gloves in covered container, according to facility policy.						
5. Washes hands (or uses alcohol hand cleaner).						

Passed Skill ________ Failed Skill ________

______________________________ ____________
Instructor Signature Date

______________________________ ____________
Student Signature Date

PERFORMANCE REVIEW CHECKLIST

Procedure 3
Procedure: Emergency Care for Vomiting and Aspiration
Name of Nutrition Assistant ______________________
Date(s) of Program _______________ to ______________ Total number of hours satisfactorily completed _________
Social Security # or Other Identifying Information of Nutrition Assistant ______________________________
Program Code Number (if any) ____________ S = Satisfactory Performance U = Unsatisfactory Performance
Place a full signature to correspond with each set of initials appearing below:

INITIALS	CORRESPONDING SIGNATURE OF INSTRUCTOR	TITLE

PROCEDURE GUIDELINES	S/U	DATE	INITIALS	S/U	DATE	INITIALS
1. Stays with resident and calls for help.						
2. Applies gloves and other protective apparel, as needed.						
3. Keeps resident's head elevated.						
4. Keeps resident's body or head turned to side to allow fluids to drain from mouth.						
5. Provides emesis basin, plastic bag, or other container if the resident is vomiting.						
6. Notifies nurse immediately if resident: • is choking or unable to swallow • is unable to spit out vomitus, blood, or secretions in mouth						
7. If resident begins choking and airway obstruction occurs, follows procedure for clearing obstructed airway.						
8. Follows nurse's instructions when he or she arrives.						
9. Observes for and reports to nurse difficulty swallowing, bleeding, vomiting, choking, or aspiration. • Does not discard vomitus until the nurse has seen it and obtained a specimen, if needed.						
10. Disposes of items containing blood or other body secretions according to facility policy.						
11. Removes gloves and disposes according to facility policy.						
12. Washes hands (or uses alcohol hand cleaner).						

Passed Skill __________ Failed Skill __________

______________________________________ ______________
Instructor Signature Date

______________________________________ ______________
Student Signature Date

PERFORMANCE REVIEW CHECKLIST

Procedure 4
Procedure: Emergency Care for Clearing the Obstructed Airway in a Conscious Adult Who is Sitting or Standing
Name of Nutrition Assistant ____________________
Date(s) of Program ______________ to ______________ Total number of hours satisfactorily completed ________
Social Security # or Other Identifying Information of Nutrition Assistant ____________________
Program Code Number (if any) __________ S = Satisfactory Performance U = Unsatisfactory Performance
Place a full signature to correspond with each set of initials appearing below:

INITIALS	CORRESPONDING SIGNATURE OF INSTRUCTOR	TITLE

PROCEDURE GUIDELINES	S/U	DATE	INITIALS	S/U	DATE	INITIALS
1. Asks resident, "Are you choking?" or "Can you speak?"						
2. If resident can speak or cough, leaves alone and observes to see if he or she can cough obstruction out. Assists if cough is weak and ineffective or resident is in obvious distress.						
3. Stays with resident and calls for help.						
4. Tells resident he or she will help.						
5. Stands behind resident and wraps arms around waist.						
6. Makes a fist with one hand and places thumb side against abdomen, just above the navel.						
7. Grasps fist with opposite hand. Avoids pressing on ribs or breastbone with forearms.						
8. Squeezes inward and upward five times. Each thrust is a separate and distinct movement with the intent of removing the obstruction.						
9. If resident does not expel foreign body, repeats inward, upward thrusts. If resident begins to cough forcefully, waits to see if object is expelled.						
10. Repeats abdominal thrusts until object is expelled or resident loses consciousness. Activates EMS system, if this has not already been done. (Sends someone else, if possible. Remains with resident and continues to relieve obstruction.)						
11. When foreign body is expelled, stays with resident and follows nurse's directions.						
12. Washes hands (or uses alcohol hand cleaner).						

Passed Skill __________ Failed Skill __________

______________________________ ______________
Instructor Signature Date

______________________________ ______________
Student Signature Date

PERFORMANCE REVIEW CHECKLIST

Procedure 5

Procedure: Feeding the Dependent Resident

Name of Nutrition Assistant ______________________

Date(s) of Program ______________ to ______________ Total number of hours satisfactorily completed ________

Social Security # or Other Identifying Information of Nutrition Assistant ______________________________

Program Code Number (if any) ____________ S = Satisfactory Performance U = Unsatisfactory Performance

Place a full signature to correspond with each set of initials appearing below:

INITIALS	CORRESPONDING SIGNATURE OF INSTRUCTOR	TITLE

PROCEDURE GUIDELINES	S/U	DATE	INITIALS	S/U	DATE	INITIALS
1. Washes hands (or uses alcohol hand cleaner).						
2. Prepares resident and obtains tray. • Applies clothing protector. • Wipes resident's hands, if needed. • Identifies correct resident. • Checks food items on tray against tray card and type of diet.						
3. Places tray on table. Sits at or below resident's eye level.						
4. Offers resident water or cool liquid to moisten the mouth and throat and tests ability to swallow. • Follows care plan for giving liquids. Uses a straw, if resident able.						
5. Informs resident what is on the tray and asks what he or she would like to eat first.						
6. Fills fork or spoon half full. • If resident has not requested a specific food item first, informs resident what food is on the utensil. • Using spoon (utensil), applies gentle downward pressure on lips or tip of tongue if resident does not respond by opening mouth. • If resident has had a stroke, places food in unaffected side of the mouth.						
7. Alternates liquids and solids. • Paces feeding to allow resident time to chew and swallow safely.						
8. Converses with resident during meal.						
9. Wipes resident's mouth and hands as needed.						
10. Removes tray when resident has finished.						
11. Washes resident's hands and face, if necessary.						
12. Removes clothing protector.						
13. Removes food from clothing or wheelchair, if needed.						
14. Removes tray.						
15. Washes hands (or uses alcohol hand cleaner).						
16. Accurately records appetite and fluid intake.						

Passed Skill __________ Failed Skill __________

______________________________________ ______________

Instructor Signature Date

______________________________________ ______________

Student Signature Date

PERFORMANCE REVIEW CHECKLIST

Procedure 6
Procedure: Measuring Fluid Intake
Name of Nutrition Assistant ______________________
Date(s) of Program ______________ to ______________ Total number of hours satisfactorily completed ________
Social Security # or Other Identifying Information of Nutrition Assistant ______________________________
Program Code Number (if any) ____________ S = Satisfactory Performance U = Unsatisfactory Performance
Place a full signature to correspond with each set of initials appearing below:

INITIALS	CORRESPONDING SIGNATURE OF INSTRUCTOR	TITLE

PROCEDURE GUIDELINES	S/U	DATE	INITIALS	S/U	DATE	INITIALS
1. Washes hands (or uses alcohol hand cleaner).						
2. Gathers supplies: • graduate or measuring container • I&O record • equivalent list, if equivalents not listed on I&O record • pen • scratch paper, if needed • calculator, if needed						
3. Estimates or measures and records all fluid consumed by the resident.						
4. Checks all serving containers for remaining liquid.						
5. Determines amount of each serving from the equivalent list.						
6. Accurately estimates (or measures) the amount of liquid remaining.						
7. Subtracts the amount remaining from amount of serving to determine fluid intake.						
8. Accurately records time and amount of fluid intake on the I&O record.						
9. Washes hands (or uses alcohol hand cleaner).						

Passed Skill __________ Failed Skill __________

______________________________________ ______________
Instructor Signature Date

______________________________________ ______________
Student Signature Date

PERFORMANCE REVIEW CHECKLIST

Procedure 7
Procedure: Serving Fresh Drinking Water
Name of Nutrition Assistant ______________________
Date(s) of Program ______________ to ______________ Total number of hours satisfactorily completed _________
Social Security # or Other Identifying Information of Nutrition Assistant ______________________________
Program Code Number (if any) ___________ S = Satisfactory Performance U = Unsatisfactory Performance
Place a full signature to correspond with each set of initials appearing below:

INITIALS	CORRESPONDING SIGNATURE OF INSTRUCTOR	TITLE

PROCEDURE GUIDELINES	S/U	DATE	INITIALS	S/U	DATE	INITIALS
1. Obtains lists of residents with special fluid orders and preferences, such as NPO or no ice.						
2. Washes hands (or uses alcohol hand cleaner).						
3. Gathers supplies on clean utility cart. • container of clean ice • clean ice scoop in plastic bag or covered container • large plastic trash bag attached to side of cart and hanging open to catch falling ice • pitcher of clean water (or fills pitchers at sink, according to facility policy) • extra cups and straws						
4. Pushes cart down hallway. Stops at each room. • Knocks on each door and waits for response. • Identifies self, greets resident(s), identifies each resident and explains procedure. • Checks and follows list of special fluid orders and resident preferences for ice, straws. • Refills pitchers, one at a time.						
5. Empties and rinses one pitcher at the sink.						
6. Takes pitcher to cart in hallway. Fills with ice. • Holds pitcher over open plastic bag while adding ice. • Keeps scoop covered when not in use. • Ice is not contaminated by touching hands, outside of cooler, etc. Uses good infection control technique to avoid contamination.						
7. Fills pitcher with clean water from pitcher or sink.						
8. Returns pitchers to correct resident.						
9. Provides clean straw and cup, if needed.						
10. Offers and pours glass of water for each resident and encourages fluid intake. Assists, if needed. • If a resident is assisted, washes hands (or uses alcohol hand cleaner) before continuing.						
11. Records fluid intake on I&O record, if ordered.						
12. Returns cart and supplies to proper storage area.						
13. Washes hands (or uses alcohol hand cleaner).						

Passed Skill __________ Failed Skill __________

______________________________ ______________
Instructor Signature Date

______________________________ ______________
Student Signature Date

PERFORMANCE REVIEW CHECKLIST

Procedure Number
Procedure: ____________________
Name of Nutrition Assistant ____________________
Date(s) of Program __________ to __________ Total number of hours satisfactorily completed __________
Social Security # or Other Identifying Information of Nutrition Assistant ____________________
Program Code Number (if any) __________ S = Satisfactory Performance U = Unsatisfactory Performance
Place a full signature to correspond with each set of initials appearing below:

INITIALS	CORRESPONDING SIGNATURE OF INSTRUCTOR	TITLE

PROCEDURE GUIDELINES	S/U	DATE	INITIALS	S/U	DATE	INITIALS

Passed Skill __________ Failed Skill __________

____________________ ____________
Instructor Signature Date

____________________ ____________
Student Signature Date

PERFORMANCE REVIEW CHECKLIST

Procedure Number

Procedure: ____________________

Name of Nutrition Assistant ____________________

Date(s) of Program __________ to __________ Total number of hours satisfactorily completed __________

Social Security # or Other Identifying Information of Nutrition Assistant ____________________

Program Code Number (if any) __________ S = Satisfactory Performance U = Unsatisfactory Performance

Place a full signature to correspond with each set of initials appearing below:

INITIALS	CORRESPONDING SIGNATURE OF INSTRUCTOR	TITLE

PROCEDURE GUIDELINES	S/U	DATE	INITIALS	S/U	DATE	INITIALS

Passed Skill __________ Failed Skill __________

____________________ ____________________

Instructor Signature Date

____________________ ____________________

Student Signature Date

PERFORMANCE REVIEW CHECKLIST

Procedure Number
Procedure: ______________________________
Name of Nutrition Assistant ____________________
Date(s) of Program ____________ to ____________ Total number of hours satisfactorily completed ________
Social Security # or Other Identifying Information of Nutrition Assistant ______________________
Program Code Number (if any) __________ S = Satisfactory Performance U = Unsatisfactory Performance
Place a full signature to correspond with each set of initials appearing below:

INITIALS	CORRESPONDING SIGNATURE OF INSTRUCTOR	TITLE

PROCEDURE GUIDELINES	S/U	DATE	INITIALS	S/U	DATE	INITIALS

Passed Skill ________ Failed Skill ________

______________________________ ____________
Instructor Signature Date

______________________________ ____________
Student Signature Date

PERFORMANCE REVIEW CHECKLIST

Procedure Number

Procedure: ______________________________

Name of Nutrition Assistant ____________________

Date(s) of Program ______________ to ______________ Total number of hours satisfactorily completed __________

Social Security # or Other Identifying Information of Nutrition Assistant ____________________________

Program Code Number (if any) __________ S = Satisfactory Performance U = Unsatisfactory Performance

Place a full signature to correspond with each set of initials appearing below:

INITIALS	CORRESPONDING SIGNATURE OF INSTRUCTOR	TITLE

PROCEDURE GUIDELINES	S/U	DATE	INITIALS	S/U	DATE	INITIALS

Passed Skill __________ Failed Skill __________

______________________________ ______________

Instructor Signature Date

______________________________ ______________

Student Signature Date

PERFORMANCE REVIEW CHECKLIST

Procedure Number

Procedure: ______________________________

Name of Nutrition Assistant ____________________

Date(s) of Program ____________ to ____________ Total number of hours satisfactorily completed ________

Social Security # or Other Identifying Information of Nutrition Assistant ________________________

Program Code Number (if any) ________ S = Satisfactory Performance U = Unsatisfactory Performance

Place a full signature to correspond with each set of initials appearing below:

INITIALS	CORRESPONDING SIGNATURE OF INSTRUCTOR	TITLE

PROCEDURE GUIDELINES	S/U	DATE	INITIALS	S/U	DATE	INITIALS

Passed Skill ________ Failed Skill ________

______________________________ ____________

Instructor Signature Date

______________________________ ____________

Student Signature Date

PERFORMANCE REVIEW CHECKLIST

Procedure Number

Procedure: ______________________________

Name of Nutrition Assistant ____________________

Date(s) of Program ____________ to ____________ Total number of hours satisfactorily completed ________

Social Security # or Other Identifying Information of Nutrition Assistant ______________________________

Program Code Number (if any) __________ S = Satisfactory Performance U = Unsatisfactory Performance

Place a full signature to correspond with each set of initials appearing below:

INITIALS	CORRESPONDING SIGNATURE OF INSTRUCTOR	TITLE

PROCEDURE GUIDELINES	S/U	DATE	INITIALS	S/U	DATE	INITIALS

Passed Skill ________ Failed Skill ________

Instructor Signature ______________________________ Date ____________

Student Signature ______________________________ Date ____________

GLOSSARY

abuse—illegal activities, such as willful infliction of injury, unreasonable confinement, intimidation, threats, or punishment. Abuse results in physical harm, pain, or mental anguish.

accidents—unexpected events that often result in injuries, which can range from minor to serious.

adaptive devices—equipment and utensils used to promote independence by changing the way a task is done.

airborne route—pathogens enter the air in respiratory secretions.

antecedent—an event that causes or triggers a behavior.

antibiotics—medications used to eliminate certain types of infections.

antiseptic—a product used to cleanse the skin and as a scrub to remove microorganisms before certain invasive procedures.

aspiration—a serious condition in which food, water, or other objects accidentally enter the trachea and lungs.

attending behavior—body language that shows that you are alert and interested in the message being communicated.

bacteria—microorganisms that can be eliminated with antibiotics.

barrier—something that interferes with communication.

calorie-controlled diets—balanced diets served to residents who are overweight.

carbohydrates—food products that provide fuel and energy for the body.

chain of infection—six factors necessary for an infection to develop.

chemicals—substances that may be harmful if they touch the skin or mucous membranes, are swallowed, or are inhaled. Most cleaning products are chemicals.

clear liquid diet—a diet that is high in water and carbohydrates and consists of liquids that you can see through.

cognitive impairment—a decline in intellectual functioning.

common vehicle—spread of infection through items that we ingest, such as food, water, or medications.

consequences—the outcome of a behavior.

consistent—all staff use the same approaches when caring for the resident.

dentures—false teeth.

diabetic diet—a diet served to residents with diabetes mellitus.

diet card—a plastic card or paper printed on a computer that lists the resident's name, room number, and type of diet. Food allergies, preferences, dislikes, and adaptive devices may be included as well.

direct contact—touching an infected person, such as when shaking hands.

disinfection—processes used to destroy pathogens in the environment with a chemical or cleaning agent.

droplet method—spreading pathogens through respiratory secretions. Pathogens spread by droplets usually do not travel more than 3 feet from the infected person.

dysphagia—difficulty swallowing food and liquids because of a medical problem.

edema—swelling of the body.

empathy—understanding how the resident feels without feeling it for him or with him. It is connecting with, and supporting a resident when he or she works through difficult times.

epiglottis—a small, muscular flap that covers the trachea when you swallow to prevent food and liquid from entering the lungs.

factual—information that you *know* is true, not what you *think* may have happened.

fats—food products such as butter and oil, which are used as a source of energy and heat.

feedback—confirmation that the message was received as intended; it may be verbal or nonverbal.

fluid restrictions—a limitation on the total liquid allowed in a 24-hour period.

fluid intake—all liquid that the resident takes into the body on a given day.

food pyramid—a chart developed by the U.S. Department of Agriculture to provide an easy-to-understand picture of daily nutritional requirements.

force fluids—an expression that means to encourage a resident to drink as many fluids as possible.

full liquid diet—A diet consisting of all clear liquids plus milk-based liquids.

good body mechanics—using the largest, strongest muscles to do the job.

hand-over-hand technique—placing your hand over the resident's hand and guiding him or her to perform the desired action.

Health Insurance Portability and Accountability Act (HIPAA)—laws governing privacy, confidentiality, medical records, and release of resident information.

hemianopsia—a condition in which the resident has blindness in half the visual field.

identification band—a plastic band placed around the wrist or ankle listing identifying information.

incident—an occurrence that disrupts the normal procedures and routine of the facility.

indirect contact—touching environmental surfaces and objects such as soiled linen, supplies, equipment, counter tops, door knobs, or faucets that have unseen pathogens on them.

infection—a state of illness caused by foreign organisms (pathogens) in the body.

infection control—practices that prevent the spread of infection.

intake and output (I&O)—monitoring all liquid taken in and put out by a resident each day.

lactose intolerance—the inability to properly digest milk sugar (lactose).

lethargy—abnormal drowsiness.

licensed practical nurse (LPN)/licensed vocational nurse (LVN)—a nurse who has completed one year to 18 months of full-time nursing education and has passed a state licensing examination. In Texas and California, these nurses are called LVNs. Other states use the LPN designation.

lockout-tagout—a system in which a locking device is placed on a broken electrical or mechanical item in a way that prevents it from being used.

low-fat and low-cholesterol diets—diets served to residents with heart, blood vessel, liver, and gallbladder disease in which fats are limited or avoided.

malnutrition—inadequate nutrition due to poor diet or inability to absorb nutrients.

material safety data sheets (MSDS)—forms that provide information and instructions for safe use, health risks, first aid, and safety precautions for using chemicals.

mechanical soft diet—a diet served to residents with chewing problems in which meats and hard foods are ground to the consistency of hamburger. Soft items, such as bread, are not ground.

mechanically altered diets—chopped or blenderized diets served to residents who have chewing, swallowing, or digestive disorders.

message—the information the sender wants to communicate.

microorganisms/microbes—living organisms that are present everywhere in the environment that cannot be seen with the eye.

milliliters (mL)/cubic centimeters (cc)—metric units of measure; two equivalent measurements used for monitoring and documenting intake and output.

minerals—an essential part of all cells that contribute to the formation of the bones, teeth, and nails, and help rebuild body tissues.

mode of transmission—the method by which a disease is spread.

neglect—deliberate or accidental failure to provide needed care or services.

no concentrated sweets diet—a diet served to diabetics in which only concentrated sweets, such as sugar, canned fruits, and sweetened desserts, are restricted.

normal flora—healthy microbes that are helpful to the function of the body.

nourishments—*substantial* food items given to selected residents to increase nutrient intake. They are usually *planned and ordered by the facility dietitian* and include foods such as sandwiches, instant breakfast, milkshakes, pudding, whole milk, yogurt, cottage cheese, and ice cream.

NPO—the medical abbreviation for "nothing by mouth."

nursing assistant—the health care team member who provides most of the personal care to the residents. The assistant must pass a state-approved class and written and skills test.

nutrients—chemical substances in food that are necessary for life.

nutrition assistant—a care worker who has successfully completed a state-approved class. He or she may assist certain residents with food and fluids.

objective—factual observations that can be observed by others by seeing, hearing, feeling, touching, and smelling.

OBRA—the abbreviation for the *Omnibus Budget Reconciliation Act*. The OBRA legislation of 1987 governs long-term care today.

obstructed airway—a serious condition in which the airway is blocked by food or a foreign object.

open-ended questions—questions that are worded in a way to give you insight into what the resident thinks and feels.

paraphrasing—a means of showing that you understand what has been said.

pathogens—microbes that cause disease.

personal protective equipment (PPE)—garments and apparel that protect the health care worker from contracting a disease from a resident. PPE also protects the resident from contracting a disease from a microbe passed from the worker's hands or uniform.

portal of entry—the place in the body where microbes enter the body.

portal of exit—how the pathogens leave the body, such as in urine, stool, blood, body fluids, secretions, excretions, or droplets.

protected health information (PHI)—identifying information, such as name, admission and discharge dates, phone numbers, or pictures.

proteins—nature's building blocks that are essential for growth, healing, and good health.

pureed diet—a diet blended with liquid so the food is smooth without large particles. The food for a normal pureed diet is the consistency of pudding or baby food, is not watery, and will support an upright plastic spoon.

RACE system—an abbreviation for the steps that should be followed in case of fire.

receiver—the person for whom the communication is intended.

registered nurse (RN)—a nurse who has completed two to four years of nursing education and passed a state licensing examination.

regular diet—a normal, unrestricted diet that is well balanced and has a variety of foods from the food pyramid.

reservoir—the place where pathogens live and grow.

Residents' Bill of Rights—part of the nursing home law that guarantees residents the same rights as any other citizen of the United States.

resolved—a resident is stable and out of danger following an incident or medical problem.

risk factors—conditions that suggest a problem may develop. Identifying risk factors and planning preventive care are key nursing functions. The presence of a risk factor does not mean a complication will develop. Once the risk is known, nursing personnel plan care designed to reduce or minimize the risk, thus preventing the complication.

sender—the person who originates communication.

snacks—*light foods* that are *given to any resident* between meals and at bedtime. Snacks include items such as graham crackers, fruit, and cookies.

sodium-restricted diets—diets served to residents with heart or kidney disease. The amount of sodium (salt) permitted each day is ordered by the doctor.

soft or **bland diets**—served to residents with digestive problems, and others who cannot eat spiced or seasoned food. Seasoning is limited and the residue is low.

source—the germ that causes disease.

standard precautions—methods used by health care workers to prevent the spread of infection.

standards of care—accepted, common health care practices based on many sources of information, including government agencies, laws such as the residents' rights document, current information about health care, publications, and facility policies.

sterilization—eliminating all microbes by using heat, gas, or chemicals.

strict I&O—a precise method of monitoring all liquid taken in and put out by a resident each day.

subjective—observations that may or may not be factual. Subjective observations are based on what you think or information the resident gives you that may or may not be true.

supplements—usually *liquid nutritional products* or puddings that are ordered by the physician for *specific residents* to promote weight gain or to correct a specific medical problem. Supplements are given to make up for a deficiency, strengthen the whole, or promote healing.

susceptible host—the person who can contract an infection. People who are very young, very old, have certain diseases, or use poor infection control practices are very susceptible.

sympathy—feeling very sorry for someone because of her or his physical condition or situation. Feeling sympathetic involves accepting others' feelings as your own. This is a negative emotion that should be avoided.

therapeutic diets—planned by the dietitian to treat certain medical diseases or conditions.

thermal burns—burns caused by contact with a hot substance, object, or open flame.

universal choking sign—putting one or both hands about the throat.

viruses—tiny pathogens that cause many diseases and cannot be eliminated by antibiotics.

vitamins—organic compounds found in foods that perform vital functions and regulate processes in the body.

water—an essential nutrient for life and health; water makes up 80% of body weight in infants. By late adulthood, approximately 40% of body weight is water. Water is important for maintaining fluid balance, preserving essential minerals, and preventing major organ failure.

INDEX